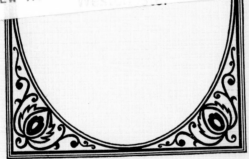

Nutrition
in a Nutshell

The proof of the pudding is in the eating
and in the subsequent metabolic effects.

The Author

It can safely be said that no one has deeper insight or is more qualified to write on the subject of nutrition than Roger J. Williams. He is the discoverer of pantothenic acid, a key B vitamin required in the machinery of all oxygen-using organisms, and did pioneer work with folic acid, an anti-anemia vitamin, and gave it its name. Since 1941, Professor Williams has been Director of the Clayton Foundation Biochemical Institute at the University of Texas, where more vitamins and their variants have been discovered than in any other laboratory in the world.

Born in India in 1893, the son of missionary parents, he received his B.S. degree from the University of Redlands and his M.S. and Ph.D. degrees from the University of Chicago. As early as 1919, when nutritional science was a mere infant, he was teaching medical students in the University of Chicago about nutrition and writing his doctoral thesis on the nutrition of yeast cells and their vitamin needs. Ever since, at the University of Oregon, Oregon State University, and the University of Texas, he has been exploring in the field of nutrition and has played a substantial role in bringing our knowledge of nutrition—including man's nutrition—to its present advanced and forward-looking state.

Long recognized by fellow scientists as a leader in nutrition and biochemistry, Professor Williams is a member of numerous scholarly and scientific organizations. In 1946, he was elected to membership in the select National Academy of Sciences. He also received the Mead Johnson Award of the American Institute of Nutrition and honorary degrees from Redlands, Columbia, and Oregon State University.

His broad knowledge has been utilized in connection with his membership on the medical boards of the National Polio Foundation, the Multiple Sclerosis Society, and the Muscular Dystrophy Associations of America, Inc., as a consultant for the American Cancer Society, and as a member of the National Food and Nutrition Board.

In 1957, he became President of the American Chemical Society, the largest scientific organization in the world. He is the only biochemist who has been so honored.

NUTRITION IN A NUTSHELL

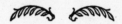

Roger J. Williams

With illustrations by Nell Taylor

Doubleday & Company, Inc., Garden City, New York

This book is dedicated
to my eldest brother
ROBERT R. WILLIAMS
a world leader in the
promotion of better nutrition

Acknowledgments

I should like to acknowledge with grateful appreciation the help of those who have read the manuscript of *Nutrition in a Nutshell* during the various stages of its preparation and who have offered suggestions and/or encouragement. Among these are my colleagues: Robert E. Eakin*, Margaret A. Eppright*, James B. Gilbert†, C. Richard King, T. S. Painter*, Richard B. Pelton, Lester J. Reed*, Lorene L. Rogers*, William Shive*, D. J. Sibley, Jr.†, Frank L. Siegel*, Alfred Taylor*, George W. Watt*, Daniel M. Ziegler*, and M. Phyllis Williams, my wife. Others located elsewhere who have given similar help are Walter C. Alvarez†, Edward L. Bortz†, Vernon Cheldelin*, Conrad A. Elvehjem*, E. E. Howe*, Ralph W. Gerard*†, Grace A. Goldsmith†, Robert S. Goodhart†, Wendell Griffith*, C. Glen King*, Chauncey Leake*, O. Lee Kline*, Herbert E. Longenecker*, Lloyd C. Miller*, Irvine H. Page†, H. R. Rosenberg*, W. Henry Sebrell†, Fredrick J. Stare*†, Roger W. Truesdail*, R. R. Williams*, and Lemuel D. Wright*.

None of these individuals should be held responsible for what is in the final copy. A few of them (but very few) would

* These individuals hold nonmedical doctorate degrees (usually the Ph.D. degree).

† These individuals hold M.D. degrees.

differ from me on some substantial points. The comments of all have been carefully weighed.

I wish particularly to acknowledge the help of my secretary, Alice M. Timmerman, whose expertness and devotion to her job has engendered admiration on the part of all who know her. .

Roger J. Williams

Contents

Preface

The whole story of nutrition, with or without a happy ending, cannot be told yet because it is still unfolding. Week by week, year by year, and decade by decade, new clues are coming to light in the research laboratories of the world.

The story becomes more interesting as new clues develop. It is ten times more intriguing now than it was when middle-aged practicing physicians heard it in their medical-school days. It promises to be more thrilling a decade from now.

As a biochemist I have been in the midst of this story since the very early chapters. When nutritional science was in its infancy I helped teach medical students in the University of Chicago what was then known about the subject. Since then I have been for decades actively and continuously engaged in exploring, discovering, and developing better insights into nutrition and its meaning.

The time has come for one who can present a firsthand rather than a second- or thirdhand account to tell the story of nutrition to nonscientists who are not interested in the technicalities of biochemistry. Nutrition is at the threshold of new and revolutionary developments and its potentialities for the improvement of health are vast.

The general story—beginning at the beginning—has never been told in this form before. The approach is fresh and the point of view forward looking. While expert nutritionists and physicians may well ponder over the contents of this little book, it is being written primarily for the public, each of whom has a stake in the outcome.

There exists for each individual a personal story of his own nutrition which he may be able to modify or even revolutionize. Whether this story can be manipulated to yield a happy ending depends in part on his own understanding and insight into what nutrition is all about. Understanding and insight are one's only protection against those who, on the one hand, may regard nutrition as a science completely wrapped up twenty years ago, or on the other hand, against those who make extravagant and ignorant claims for their own faddist notions.

Roger J. Williams

Nutrition
in a Nutshell

I

When Does Nutrition Start?

At that dramatic moment when a microscopic wiggly male cell pushes its way into a much larger egg cell and joins forces with it, a human being begins to exist, and nutrition starts.

This developmental period, when things can definitely go "right" or "wrong," is vitally important, and nutrition can exert a profound influence that is felt throughout life. The growing embryo which becomes organized to an unbelievable degree, cannot be produced from nothing; it must get its sustenance hour by hour and day by day from the mother—who in turn gets from the food that she eats everything that she passes on to her child-to-be.

If the mother is not completely healthy and well nourished in every respect, she may fail to furnish the embryo with the best nutrition. In this case all sorts of difficulties—major or minor—may arise depending upon what nutritional items are in short supply and how great are the shortages. Deformities, stillbirths, retarded mental development, miscarriages and other more obscure troubles that show up in later life may have their origin in improper embryonic nutrition.

The story of human nutrition contains many blank pages because experimentation must be limited. No scientist will deliberately starve or partially starve an unborn baby in order to find out what troubles will develop later in life! Experiments of this sort can be done with animals which, for pur-

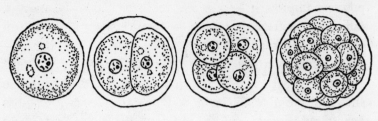

THE FIRST 4 DAYS OF HUMAN DEVELOPMENT
MICROSCOPIC VIEW (x 100)

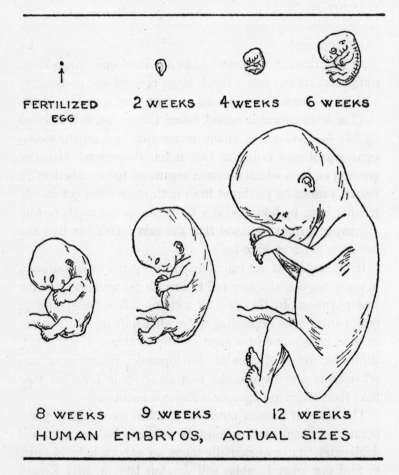

FERTILIZED EGG　　2 WEEKS　　4 WEEKS　　6 WEEKS

8 WEEKS　　9 WEEKS　　12 WEEKS
HUMAN EMBRYOS, ACTUAL SIZES

It is during embryonic development that nutrition starts.

poses of improving human life, are expendable. In animals, difficulties in great variety and of extreme severity can be produced at will merely by furnishing—through the mothers—faulty nutrition to the growing embryos.

Various stages in the development of a human being are shown in the illustrations on page 2. After the male cell has penetrated the egg cell, the fertilized egg is large enough to be visible to the naked eye. Just barely, however, as it has a diameter less than that of an ordinary pin. To show more what it looks like and how it develops during the first four days, pictures are shown (p. 2) enlarged 100 times. The *actual* sizes and appearance of the embryos in later weeks are shown in the lower illustrations on the same page.

But this gives only a gross picture. When the original fertilized egg cell divides and subdivides, the "daughter" cells are at first almost duplicates of the original parent cell. Before many generations have been produced, the daughter cells begin looking more and more like "adopted" daughters and before long they lose all resemblance to the original parent. Some become bone cells, some muscle cells, some nerve cells, some skin cells, some blood cells; hundreds of different kinds of cells develop and often billions of each kind.

This mysterious process of becoming different is little understood. Biologists appropriately call it "differentiation."

The almost unbelievable lengths to which the differentness extends is made clear in the pictures of twenty different human cells, (pp. 4, 5) all magnified to exactly the same degree (× 200). The smallest cell shown, even when magnified to this extent, appears smaller than a birdshot, while the largest appears enormous by comparison. A motor nerve cell appears like a string 600 feet long with a frayed "knot" on one end about the size of a marble. A skeletal muscle cell on the same scale is often about the size and shape of a 200-foot-long pencil. Tremendous variation in form is also shown. Some

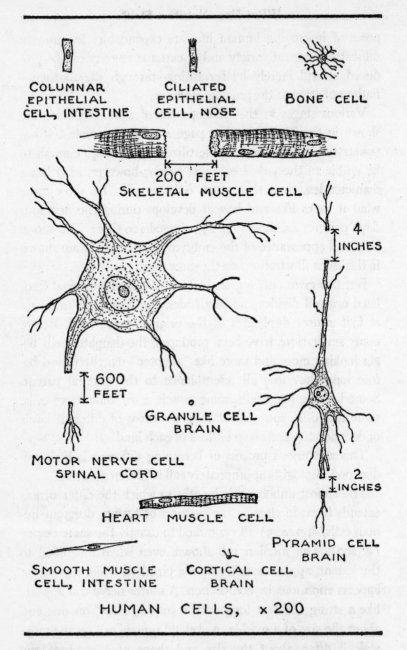

COLUMNAR
EPITHELIAL
CELL, INTESTINE

CILIATED
EPITHELIAL
CELL, NOSE

BONE CELL

200 FEET
SKELETAL MUSCLE CELL

4
INCHES

600
FEET

GRANULE CELL
BRAIN

MOTOR NERVE CELL
SPINAL CORD

2
INCHES

HEART MUSCLE CELL

PYRAMID CELL
BRAIN

SMOOTH MUSCLE
CELL, INTESTINE

CORTICAL CELL
BRAIN

HUMAN CELLS, × 200

Each of twenty types of cells represented in the illustrations above
and on the facing page (as well as many more types) needs day-to-day

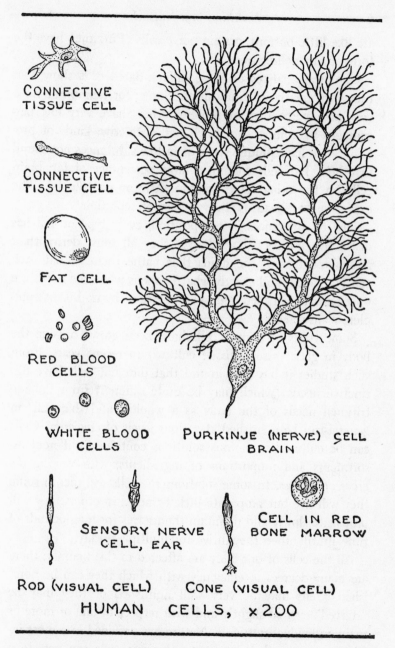

CONNECTIVE
TISSUE CELL

CONNECTIVE
TISSUE CELL

FAT CELL

RED BLOOD
CELLS

WHITE BLOOD
CELLS

PURKINJE (NERVE) CELL
BRAIN

SENSORY NERVE
CELL, EAR

CELL IN RED
BONE MARROW

ROD (VISUAL CELL)

CONE (VISUAL CELL)

HUMAN CELLS, x200

adequate nutrition. Each type probably has a set of needs which is
quantitatively if not qualitatively distinctive.

are like little buttons; certain nerve cells (Purkinje) have the form of a branching tree.

Chemical analyses of these differentiated cells show that they vary greatly in composition. Some, for example, have a very high percentage of protein, others have very low percentages by comparison. Each has distinctive kinds of protein. Some have unique types of fatlike substances not found in others. Fat cells contain a large percentage of fat; brain cells on the other hand contain little or no true fat. The expression "fat head" is always a misrepresentation.

Due to differences in composition, every type of cell has distinctive nutritional needs, yet they all must derive their nourishment from the fluids that bathe them. What each cell type needs and exactly what happens when the needs are only partially satisfied, are open questions by no means completely answered.

Some types of human cells have been grown outside the body in glass vessels (tissue culture) in recent years. From such studies it has been found that different cells have distinctive needs (which may be quite different from the nutritional needs of the body as a whole), and that cells in general can be nourished at various levels of efficiency. Cells can be cultured in various solutions containing different assortments and proportions of ingredients, with *varying degrees of success*. In some solutions the cells will die; in some they will live but propagate little or none; in others they will propagate slowly and maintain themselves for long periods of time, in still others they thrive and multiply readily.

All the cells of our body are affected in this manner; there are many degrees of efficiency with which they can be nourished. Cells may be very well nourished or they may be "starved" ever so slightly and with respect to one or more of many individual nutrients. Nature has provided in a most intricate manner that growing embryonic cells can get—to a reasonably satisfactory degree—everything they need, provided the mother eats wisely. If she tries to subsist on doughnuts and coffee, the embryonic cells are bound to be starved in many ways.

Perfect cellular nutrition throughout our whole bodies, in the sense that every cell gets exactly what it needs for maximum efficiency, is probably as rare as perfect health or as perfect human conduct. To err is human, but this does not make it desirable to make as many errors as possible. Mothers-to-be need to be nourished with more than ordinary care if the cells which make up the growing embryo are furnished nutrition at a *high level* of efficiency.

II

What Needs Nourishment?

We sometimes jokingly say "It's time to feed our faces," when it is obvious that we mean our entire bodies (including our faces) are ready for nourishment.

Because the various parts of our body do not automatically become nourished equally well when we eat, we will get a better picture of what the nutrition of an adult is like if we look briefly at different parts of bodies that require nourishment.

We might begin anywhere in the body but there is some logic in starting with the skeleton which supports all other tissues. Superficially, our bones are largely mineral matter—mostly calcium phosphates—and one might suppose that once the skeleton is formed, nutrition of the bone could stop. This is far from true. By the use of "isotopic tracers," biochemists have found that even in an adult body, minerals are constantly leaving and entering the bones. This means that the bones are *alive*; the situation is dynamic rather than static. Bones contain living bone cells (p. 4) which require not only minerals for building bone but all of the other food elements that other living cells need in order to maintain themselves.

An emergency need for these cells arises when a bone becomes broken. If these cells had ceased to live and function when the adult skeleton became formed, a broken bone would remain broken for the rest of one's life. When a bone does become broken the nourishment of these bone cells is crucially important; they need not only the minerals required for repairing the damage but the cells themselves need to "eat" and keep well.

These bone cells, like all other cells, can be nourished at various levels of efficiency. This is related to the fact that sometimes bones knit slowly and sometimes rapidly. The rate of healing can be retarded by relatively poor nutrition of the cells that do the repair work; it can be stepped up by improving the nutrition of these cells. Competent physicians who treat fracture cases, especially those who are nutrition-minded, take pains to see that every possible measure is adopted to promote the very best nutrition possible for the bone cells.

What we have said about bone also applies to a lesser degree to teeth. Teeth are to a degree alive also, and some dynamic interchange of minerals between them and the rest of the body takes place. It is during the developmental growing stage, however, that the nourishment of the tooth-forming cells appears most important. If these cells are nourished at the highest level of excellence, they are not only furnished with adequate amounts of all the necessary raw materials for tooth building but they are furnished all the nutrients that living cells in general need in order to thrive.

That tooth-building cells can be nourished at different levels of efficiency can readily be demonstrated in experimental animals—rats, for example. When young developing rats are fed certain diets containing much sugar—and an unbalanced supply of other nutrients—they live and grow but develop unsound teeth that have a strong tendency to decay. If the same rats are fed a well-formulated diet, they not only live and grow but they develop sound teeth that do not decay. If one wishes to demonstrate the existence of different degrees of efficiency, one has only to mix—half and half—the poorer diet and the good diet. The result will be that rats eating this mixture will develop teeth intermediate in soundness; the teeth will not resist decay like those of the well-fed animals, neither will they be subject to as much decay as the teeth of the most poorly fed group.

The cells in our skin including the hair-building cells need continual nourishment; this becomes more evident and compelling when we remember that skin is constantly being worn away and replaced and hair is in the habit of growing continuously day and night, year after year.

Those who are used to handling farm animals, pets, or racing animals know that the outside appearance of the skin and hair—sleekness—is an important index of health and well being. If an animal's hair or fur is well nourished and healthy, this is an indication that the other cells of its body are at least fairly well nourished. Laboratory experience with mammals and fowls shows that many entirely different nutritional deficiencies will cause the skin and hair, or feathers, to become unhealthy and disheveled in appearance.

Physicians know the importance of a healthy skin and are often able to judge their patient's condition on this basis. Several gross vitamin deficiencies make themselves known in human beings by the unhealthy appearance of the skin. In acute adult scurvy (which is very rare*), hemorrhagic spots appear on the skin and the hair falls out; in pellagra, a rash appears on the skin whenever it is exposed to the sun or even to mild soap; in riboflavin (B_2) deficiency, inflamed areas appear on the skin at the corners of the mouth. Vitamin A deficiency results in an unhealthy skin (epithelial tissue) and a lack of resistance to infections. When any of these outward symptoms appear, they should be regarded as signals of deficiencies that are more deep-seated and probably also involve the whole biochemical mechanism of the body including many of the internal organs. Other conditions that adversely affect bodily health such as insufficiency of thyroid hormone

* Recent reports from Canada indicate that acute scurvy in infants may not be rare.

also cause the skin to become rough and unhealthy in appearance.

The tissues of the stomach and intestines need continual adequate nourishment so they can produce digestive juices and carry out the process of digestion and absorption of food materials. In the debilitating tropical disease, sprue, the difficulty lies exactly in this area. The cells and tissues that are involved in digestion and absorption become malnourished through the lack of sufficient amounts of certain vitamins, and as a result the whole body is deprived of absorbed nourishment and suffers from serious malnutrition. If the intestinal cells are furnished with the missing vitamins, they become able again to carry out their digestive and absorptive functions effectively; as a result, the devastating disease disappears and the body as a whole becomes well.

Early in the history of physiology, it was supposed that absorption which involves passage of food materials through the intestinal wall, was merely the result of a sievelike action that allowed smaller molecules to pass. More recently, however, it is clear that healthy living cells are indispensable to the complex process that often involves the intermediate chemical modification of the material which passes through. The cells carrying out this work must be kept alive and well; this can only be accomplished if they are nourished continuously at a high level of excellence.

The pancreas gland and the liver both take part in the digestion-absorption process. In order to produce all the digestive enzymes, bile acids, etc., the cells in these two organs have to be furnished all the raw materials necessary for building their products—also, these living cells, like all others in the body, must be bathed continuously in a nutrient solution that will furnish them everything they need, to live and thrive.

Constipation is often a manifestation of inadequate nutrition of the intestinal tissues. In the intestinal tract there are many involuntary "smooth" muscles which, when stimulated, cause stomach and intestinal movements. These wavelike motions keep the partially digested food moving along until the residue reaches the large bowel and is eventually eliminated. All the smooth muscles are made up of living cells which must be nourished at a high level of efficiency if the whole process is to proceed with facility and ease. In order to prevent stagnation in the intestinal tract, irritating substances (laxatives) are often used. These stimulate and drive the muscle cells, sometimes mercilessly, whereas usually all the muscle cells need in order to function well is some bulk to work on, coupled with good sound nutrition continuously furnished.

The system of arteries, veins, and capillaries which carries blood and nourishment to all parts of the body are not themselves inert pipes; their walls contain indispensable living cells which like all cells must be nourished satisfactorily in order to remain alive and well. They do not always stay well; so-called hardening of the arteries results from an unhealthy "corroded" condition which can certainly be aggravated by improper nutrition.

The center of the circulatory system—the heart—is very much alive and its continual nourishment is crucially important. It pumps blood not only all over the body, but to the heart muscle itself. This muscle utilizes a large amount of energy and the heart-muscle cells need to be "fed" a highly nutritious "diet," day in and day out. If an artery supplying blood to the heart becomes unhealthy and corroded, it is more likely to be stopped up by a small blood clot. In this case the heart-muscle cells which depend on the artery for sustenance are starved. If the starvation, particularly for oxygen, is extensive and lasts even a fraction of a minute, the victim may die of a coronary. In this case the quality of the blood may be satisfactory but if it can't get through to the heart-muscle cells, it can't carry its benefits to them. The heart cells die and, as a result, all cells in the body ultimately die.

This is another example in which failure of cells in one area to get what they need can cause severe damage elsewhere in the body.

There may be other cases in which the muscle cells of the heart are malnourished because the blood doesn't have in it the right ingredients in the right amounts. For example, several years ago when pantothenic acid was first discovered, a group of dogs was fed a diet lacking a sufficient amount of the newly discovered vitamin. They appeared outwardly satisfactory and ate the deficient diet up until a day or so before they suddenly died. Many cells and tissues had become deficient, but the dogs continued to live until the heart muscle was starved for this necessary nutrient to such an extent that it ceased to function.

There are various special organs in the body that have special and distinctive nutritional requirements. All the hormone-producing glands of the body: the thyroid gland, the pituitary, the adrenals, the sex glands, the insulin-producing cells in the pancreas, the parathyroids, are made up of living cells which, like all other living cells, need continuous and complex nourishment. In addition, these cells need the raw materials out of which the respective hormones are built.

One of these cases is particularly interesting because the hormone in question contains a specific chemical element —iodine—which is not known to be needed except as a building block for the thyroid hormone. The cells that produce the thyroid hormone are among the differentiated cells in the body; they peculiarly need iodine if they are to perform their unique function. In certain regions of the world—the Great Lakes area, the Pacific Northwest, and Switzerland are examples—iodine is at a low level in soil and vegetation. As a result, the thyroid glands of animals (dogs) and human beings are starved (relatively) for iodine; they become diseased, swell up to a large size and thus call attention to themselves (endemic goiter). They simply cannot do the job of producing the

hormone adequately unless they are furnished enough iodine
to put into it. When sufficient iodine is furnished (through
iodized salt or otherwise), the enlarged thyroid gland reduces
to normal size and the diseased condition disappears. By
limiting to different degrees the amount of iodine furnished
a mammal, it is possible to produce severe simple goiter or
any condition intermediate between this and completely
normal functioning.

The thyroid-hormone-producing cells need, of course, many
other nutrients besides iodine, and it is quite conceivable that
they might be malnourished in other ways. The iodine lack—
at different levels—is, however, relatively easily demonstrated
and hence has been brought into our discussion. There are
other diseases of the thyroid gland—those involving *over-*
activity—which cannot be cured by altering the iodine supply,
but these have origins too complicated to discuss here.

The thyroid hormone is needed all over the body; it is one
of the regulatory substances involved in stimulating the complicated chemical processes that are taking place in our bodies.
When not enough of this hormone is available, for example,
the skin becomes leathery and unhealthy in appearance. The
thyroid hormone itself may be regarded as an internally produced nutritional substance needed by the skin (and other)
cells. Indeed the thyroid hormone can be taken by mouth—
when the thyroid gland is out of order or has been mostly
removed by surgery—with the result that the skin cells and
other cells of the body obtain this needed substance from
the digested food. This is an exception—in many other cases,
introduction of hormones into the food is without effect because digestion often brings about their destruction—particularly when they are protein in nature.

Other types of cells which need very special nourishment
for reasons that are quite clear, are those contained in the
retina of the eye. The so-called visual pigments, those substances that are altered by light and thus make vision possible,

have a close relative of vitamin A in their chemical make-up. Vitamin A has to serve as a raw material for the building of visual pigments and since it cannot be made elsewhere in the body it has to be furnished in the food. The retinal cells need it in relatively large amounts and in some animals a large part of the total vitamin A in the body accumulates in these retinal cells.

To jump to the conclusion that retinal cells are the only ones that require vitamin A in their diet would be a grave mistake. For epithelial cells, which are in the skin and many places elsewhere in the body, vitamin A is a vitally important nutrient. Liver cells often contain a relative abundance of vitamin A—stored for use in other parts of the body.

Other cells that have special nutritional needs are those in the male testes that produce the sperm cells which make reproduction possible. If vitamin A is supplied in inadequate amounts to experimental animals, the males are unable to produce healthy sperm and are sterile. Females on the same deficient diet are not able to produce healthy young, even if bred to potent males. Both males and females may appear outwardly well, even though they are sterile because of inadequate nutrition.

Vitamin A is not the only nutritional element that is conspicuously necessary for reproduction. Vitamin E was initially discovered because its lack caused female rats to become sterile. Conception could take place, but the embryos did not develop; they were most often resorbed. Animals lacking sufficient vitamin E appear well and healthy in other respects. If the female rat does not become pregnant, then *apparent health* may continue.

But vitamin E is needed for purposes other than the production of healthy embryos. It is widespread in practically all the tissues of the body where it has important functions—which to date, however, are largely unknown. When a pregnant rat has insufficient vitamin E to produce a healthy litter of young, this does not mean that her body store is exhausted, it means that she doesn't have enough to take care of her own vital needs and the additional needs involved in reproduction. Her vitamin E supply can be at all levels, from abundance down to complete inadequacy.

Many essential nutrients besides vitamins A and E are needed for the production of healthy young. Because vitamin E was discovered in connection with the reproductive process in rats, there has been undue emphasis on this phase of its functioning. In rabbits, guinea pigs and rats, muscular weakness (dystrophy) and degeneration may also result from vitamin E deficiency; in chicks unhealthy blood vessels are prominent when vitamin E deficiency exists. The bodily processes in different species are sufficiently different so that a vitamin E lack might show up in a human being at quite a different place than it does in rats. Vitamin E is just as essential for human beings as it is for rats but we are not able, because dangerous experiments are out of the question, to pinpoint or demonstrate exactly where the need is most crucial. Many nutrients, including a large number we have not yet mentioned, are simultaneously necessary for the development of healthy embryos in every mammal.

The nutrition of brain and other nerve cells is unique and of great interest. When "differentiation" takes place, the cells produced are enormously different in size, shape, chemical composition, and in nutritional needs. They are also wholly different in their activity and behavior. Epithelial cells in the skin, for example, keep on multiplying and sloughing off as long as one lives. Nerve cells on the other hand cease to multiply about the time a baby is born, and the quota of brain and nerve cells does not increase during youth or adulthood.

This does not mean, of course, that brain and nerve cells loaf quiescently through life. Actually they are extremely busy in the chemical sense. Although one's brain weighs about 2 per cent as much as one's whole body, its "fuel" consumption may be up to 25 per cent of the body's total. In a small child one half of the total metabolism (chemical burning) may take place in the brain. The amount of energy that a human brain uses up in 24 hours is roughly enough to heat six quarts of water from the freezing point up to the boiling point. To have this energy available the brain needs to be supplied continuously with fuel in the form of glucose (dextrose). The brain also needs continuously the wherewithal, in the form of a large number of nutrients, to maintain itself. Nutrition of the nerve cells in the brain is sufficiently unique so that the body handles the situation differently; while most cells take their nutrition directly from the blood plasma, this is not true of the brain cells. There is what is called a "blood-brain barrier" which holds back from brain tissue higher concentrations of many of the nutrients, particularly amino acids, to which other cells and tissues have free access.

The study of the nutrition of nerve cells presents special problems because, as we have indicated, the nerve cells even during childhood do not propagate. The highly active nerve cells are known to need, however, many of the nutrients that other cells require. In various vitamin deficiencies, for example, B_1 deficiency, niacin deficiency, pantothenic acid deficiency, or vitamin B_{12} deficiency, nerve cells develop severe abnormalities in appearance and function which point unmistakably to the fact these substances are absolute necessities so far as maintaining healthy nerve cells is concerned. Also it is well known that if the thyroid hormone is not supplied to a developing brain, the child becomes an idiot.

Brain and other nerve cells are intimately concerned with many regulatory functions. In a well individual there is nervous regulation of body temperature (thermostatic control), nervous regulation of the rate of heart beat, of the breathing rate, of hormone production, and of factors that govern important phases of blood composition. Many of these regulatory processes are so vital that if they fail, immediate death may result. For carrying out all these functions nerve cells continuously need high-quality nutrition.

Another regulatory mechanism about which we will have more to say later is the complex one which makes us eat with some degree of wisdom. For example, if some self-styled food expert seeks to convince us that we need, above all things, *honey* and more *honey*, our body contains a regulatory mechanism which protects us against such foolishness. This is foolishness because honey is a very incomplete food (mostly sugars) and should be consumed sparingly. The first spoonful or two of honey may go down all right, but if one attempts to eat more and more, the body rebels; we become nauseated and if we still insist on eating more, the body, using its vomiting mechanism, may forcefully correct our intemperance.

That this regulatory mechanism also requires good nutrition to keep it in working order was shown first by Dr. Macy-Hoobler of Michigan who found that children on a well-formulated diet consumed (by choice) less candy than those on a poor diet. In our laboratories at Texas we have confirmed this finding by giving rats poor and good diets in succession and noting their voluntary consumption of sugar-water. A deficient diet causes increased consumption, while correcting the diet causes a decrease in sugar consumption. The "body wisdom" so far as eating sugar is concerned is enhanced in both children and rats by improving their nutrition. This improved nutrition has made the regulatory nerve cells more healthy and effective. Good nutrition fosters good nutrition. This reminds us of the Biblical saying "To him that hath, shall be given."

There are complex regulatory mechanisms that help guide us with respect to how much of other things we eat, such as fat. If we should go contrary to the present advice of nutritionists and decide to gulp down large quantities of fat—margarine or butter—our bodies would rebel and fat would become nauseating. There are also regulatory mechanisms that help us decide how much water to drink, how much salt to put on our food, and perhaps most important of all, *how much* energy-containing food we will eat.

All of the nerve cells involved in every one of these regulatory mechanisms (many of these cells are probably located in the hypothalamus of the brain) require good nutrition if they are going to work satisfactorily. Since cells can be nourished at various levels of efficiency, it follows that the various regulatory mechanisms can work poorly, moderately well, or extremely well, depending on the quality of the nutrition of the operating cells and tissues.

Since good nutrition fosters good nutrition, it becomes obvious why nutrition in young children is so important. If they are well nourished from the start, their regulatory mechanisms develop well, the working of their body wisdom approaches perfection, and they may go through life without ever suffering from the ills associated with malnutrition.

Every working part of our body, including all the endocrine and other regulatory mechanisms, needs good nutrition. Nature has made important provisions other than those which may be regarded body wisdom, to help us in the exceedingly complicated job of feeding at high levels of excellence every cell and tissue in our bodies. These provisions will be discussed later.

The fact that the food we eat is needed by all the cells in our bodies, coupled with the fact that all living cells require a multitude of nutrients, should make us see the folly of some of the time-honored sayings: "Iron is for the blood"; "Calcium is for bones"; "Vitamin A is for the eyes"; "Phosphorus is for the brain"; "Vitamin B_1 is for the nerves." Iron, calcium, vitamin A, phosphorus and vitamin B_1 (as well as many other nutrients to be listed in the following chapter) are each absolutely indispensable for blood *and* bones *and* eyes *and* brain *and* nerves, as well as for many, many other tissues in our bodies.

III

What Does Nourishing Food Contain?

Nutrition is like a chain in which all of the essential items are the separate links. If the chain is weak or is broken at any point the whole chain fails. If there are 40 items that are essential in the diet, and one of these is missing, nutrition fails just as truly as it would if half the links were missing. The absolute lack of any item (or of several items) results in ill health and eventually in death. An insufficient amount of any one item is enough to bring distress to the cells and tissues which are most vulnerable to this particular lack. It is not necessary that every item be furnished in required amounts at every meal or every day, because our bodies always carry some reserves. As soon as the reserves are lost, however, be they large or small, they must be replenished.

The links in the nutrition chain are chemical links. The only kind of answer to the question posed as the heading for this chapter is a chemical answer. Water is a chemical; salt is a chemical; sugar is a chemical; bread and milk are each highly complex mixtures of chemicals.

In answering the question—what does nourishing food contain?—we will be forced to give the chemical names of the individual substances that enter into our diets. There is no need whatever for the reader to become acquainted with these individual chemicals or to memorize the list, in order to take advantage of what will be said later.

In the following table are listed the more significant chemicals that enter into our daily food along with an estimate of the amounts consumed daily. This is a *selected* list of significant items; a complete list of every chemical that is present in natural food would be much longer than this. This list does not include internally produced nutrients (of which the thyroid hormone may be an example) but only the significant chemicals we consume when we eat good food.

Many of the items are listed in capital letters to indicate that they are "musts." Each of these constitutes a specific need; *no one can replace any other*, and all are required for the maintenance of the body machinery.

SIGNIFICANT CHEMICALS CONTAINED IN FOOD		ESTIMATED DAILY CONSUMPTION*
	WATER	1500. gramst
Carbohydrates etc.	Starches, sugars (glucose [dextrose], sucrose, lactose, fructose [levulose], mannose)	300. grams
	Bulk (such as cellulose and pectins)	25. grams
	Citrates, tartrates, lactates, etc.	2. grams
Fats and fatlike substances	Fats and oils (animal and vegetable sources)	85. grams
	Phospholipids	5. grams
	LINOLEIC and/or other effective unsaturated fat acids	10. grams
	Cholesterol	1. gram
Amino acids (Protein "building stones")	Glutamic acid and *glutamine*	16. grams
	LEUCINE	8. grams
	Arginine	6. grams
	Aspartic acid and *asparagin*	6. grams
	Proline	5. grams
	ISOLEUCINE	4. grams
	VALINE	4. grams
	Alanine	3. grams
	LYSINE	3. grams

	SIGNIFICANT CHEMICALS CONTAINED IN FOOD	ESTIMATED DAILY CONSUMPTION*
Amino acids (Protein "building stones")	Glycine	3. grams†
	METHIONINE	3. grams
	PHENYLALANINE	3. grams
	Serine	3. grams
	THREONINE	3. grams
	Tyrosine	3. grams
	Cystine	2. grams
	Histidine	2. grams
	TRYPTOPHANE	1. gram
Vitamins, etc.	*Inositol*	1. gram
	CHOLINE	1. gram
	VITAMIN A (different forms)	6.00 mg.
	VITAMIN D (different forms) (Sunshine can substitute)	0.040 mg.
	VITAMIN E (different forms)	6.00 mg.
	VITAMIN K (different forms)	2. mg.
	ASCORBIC ACID (C)	75. mg.
	THIAMIN (vitamin B_1)	1.5 mg.
	RIBOFLAVIN (B_2)	1.8 mg.
	PANTOTHENATE (B_3)	10. mg.
	NIACINAMIDE	15. mg.
	BIOTIN	0.2 mg.
	FOLIC ACID	1. mg.
	PYRIDOXIN (or equivalent) (B_6)	3. mg.
	COBALAMIN (B_{12})	0.002 mg. (2 mcg.)
	Rutin and related glucosides	25. mg.
	Lipoic acid	0.5 mg.
Other Chemical Elements (usually in the form of salts)	CALCIUM	750. mg.
	PHOSPHORUS (as phosphate)	750. mg.
	SODIUM	4000. mg.
	POTASSIUM	2500. mg.
	CHLORIDE	5000. mg.
	MAGNESIUM	250. mg.
	IRON	10. mg.
	ZINC	10. mg.
	MANGANESE	5. mg.
	Chromium	2. mg.

Other Chemical Elements (usually in the form of salts)	COPPER	2.	mg.†
	COBALT (in vitamin B$_{12}$; other combinations also?)	0.1	mg.
	Fluoride	0.5	mg.
	MOLYBDENUM	0.5	mg.
	Selenium	0.5	mg.
	IODIDE	0.1	mg.

---

* See page 24.

† We use here the relatively simple metric system which is uniformly used for scientific work throughout the world: One gram is approximately $\frac{1}{28}$ of an ounce; a milligram (mg.) is one thousandth of a gram; a microgram (mcg.) is one thousandth of a milligram or one millionth of a gram.

Carbohydrates and fats, for example, are not listed in capital letters because while both are highly desirable (for economic as well as other reasons) their main function is to yield energy, and energy can be obtained if necessary (expensively and not without some stress, to be sure) from amino acids or proteins. Even the glucose which we have said is necessary for brain nutrition can be produced in the body from proteins. Fats and carbohydrates needed for structural purposes also can be built from other organic food constituents.

Individual proteins are not on the list for two reasons; first, because there are too many of them to list—small amounts of hundreds of individual proteins could easily be consumed in one meal—and second, because all proteins, as we shall discuss later, yield by digestion an assortment of the amino acids listed. The nutritional value of any protein depends upon the particular assortment of these relatively few amino acids and the amounts of each it furnishes. No individual protein is needed in anyone's diet. Proteins which will yield sufficient amounts of the essential amino acids (those listed in capital letters) are needed in everyone's diet.

Certain of the items are listed in italics. This suggests that they are potentially important but that their status is uncertain. In some cases the need for an external supply exists only when, for some metabolic reason, the internal supply is limited. If this book should be revised a few years hence, it is probable that some changes would be made. Additions to the list might be made and some italicized items might be shifted to the "must" category. Nutrition and biochemistry are dynamic, developing sciences.

One item on the list—cholesterol—is not only a nonessential, but for some people it appears undesirable. It is an important constituent of our bodies, but it is manufactured within our bodies. In some individuals too much is produced; in these cases consumption of extra amounts in the food does not recommend itself on a common-sense basis. Meticulous care in the avoidance of cholesterol in the diet is, however, not warranted. We will discuss this problem later in connection with coronary heart disease.

It should be noted that after each item in the list, a definite amount is indicated. If one were to take these amounts too literally, it would be entirely misleading. On the other hand, the reason why some reasonable estimates are indicated in every case, is to emphasize the all-important *quantitative aspects of nutrition.*

Suppose, for example, we were to present a list without indicated amounts, and that some literal-minded individual should say: "All right, there are fifty-nine significant items on the list. I'll mix and consume equal amounts of each; then I'll have everything." Three dramatic things would happen to such an individual. First, he would probably go bankrupt trying to buy a day's supply on this equal-weight basis because some of the items on the list (which are needed in tiny amounts) are exceedingly costly. Second, he would choke trying to eat the dry mixture. Third, after consuming his first meal he would surely die because some of the items, like copper, cobalt and molybdenum salts, are essential in tiny amounts but are exceedingly poisonous if taken in amounts corresponding to $\frac{1}{59}$ of the weight of one meal.

The quantitative aspects of nutrition are difficult to exaggerate. Sometimes people ask: "How many vitamins do I get when I eat such and such?" As we shall make clear in later chapters, one is likely to get in a mouthful of almost any food (excluding pure sugar or starch), a few molecules at least, of most of the 59 items listed above, including most if not all of the vitamins. But a "few molecules" is like a tiny drop in a big bucket; these few would never be enough. The amount of iodine we get daily in our food if concentrated into a single speck would be barely visible, yet the number of iodine atoms it contains is about 500,000,000,000,000,000,000! Even a million million atoms of iodine would be an entirely negligible amount and if this is all we get day after day and year after year we will surely die of iodine starvation.

Whether one gets from a mouthful of food every item in about the right proportions is a serious question that usually has a negative answer. Diversification in food consumption is necessary. The quantitative aspects of nutrition are crucially important. It is not how *many* amino acids, vitamins, or minerals we get that is important. It is how *much* we get of each one. It is to emphasize this fact that *a quantity* has been designated for every item, even though the amount in each case is an estimate and allows for considerable variation as our later discussions will make clear.

Further explanation is necessary so that we can appreciate the tremendous role that proteins play in our lives and in our nutrition. A typical protein molecule may be pictured as follows: Imagine five hundred beads of twenty slightly differing shapes strung together in a definite order and then coiled and wound together in a specific manner into a spherical or elongated ball. Each bead is an amino acid (referred to previously as a protein building stone) and the whole compact complex structure is what we call a native (natural) protein molecule.

Proteins are actually highly diverse in structure; there may be, for example, more or less than 500 "beads." Beef insulin (commonly used for diabetes) is one of the simplest known proteins and has only 51 beads of 19 different kinds. Some common proteins have about 3,000 beads and some may have as many as 200,000. Proteins in general are made up of molecules which are relatively very large but still invisible.

Even without this variable number of beads, a stupendous number of proteins would be possible. It has been calculated that if there were only 12 kinds of beads to choose from and the total number of beads in proteins were always 288, there would be 100^{300} different proteins possible due to different *arrangements* of the 288 beads. This stupendous number is *much* larger than the total number of atoms in the entire earth.

One simplifying feature in protein chemistry is the fact that the beads are very limited in number (about 20) and the same identical beads enter into the make-up of all proteins. This is why in the field of nutrition we have so much to say about the beads (amino acids) and relatively little about the proteins that yield these beads on being digested.

Biochemists have shown tremendous ingenuity. Nobel Prize winning Sanger has determined, for example, the exact sequence of all the beads in insulin molecules, although of course not even insulin molecules (let alone the tinier beads) are large enough to be seen through the best microscopes. The sequences of beads in most proteins are unknown or very incompletely known.

Proteins often have "embroidered" into their structure other beads which are quite different in make-up from the amino acids. Hemoglobin of the blood, for example, has a complex structure containing iron as an intimate part of its structure; without this it could not carry oxygen to the tissues. Numerous other structures containing, for example, minerals other than iron and many of the vitamins, also enter into the make-up of many complex proteins. In considering nutritional problems, however, we often associate proteins exclusively with the constituent amino acids (beads) which are *always* present, rather than with the minerals and vitamins which are found only in particular proteins, and sometimes loosely attached.

The process of digesting a protein involves first unraveling and uncoiling the wound-up balls of bead work. This is called "denaturation" and is accomplished during cooking. If uncooked native proteins are consumed this uncoiling and unraveling must take place in the stomach and intestine preliminary to digestion.

The second step in digestion is breaking the beads apart. Our bead analogy is imperfect here because the beads are actually joined together rather than being on a string. The linkage between beads is not rigid but it is tenacious. By ordinary chemical means these beads can be wholly broken apart only by boiling the protein molecules with strong acid or alkali for about 24 hours! In biochemical work this can be done rapidly at body temperature by the use of specific catalytic agents called *enzymes*, derived from natural sources.

Enzymes are themselves proteins with distinctive embroidery (often containing minerals and/or vitamins) such that they are able for reasons incompletely understood, to hasten chemical processes. If a tiny amount of pepsin, one of the enzymes in gastric juice, is allowed to stand in the presence of egg white, the protein molecules in the egg white cease to exist; certain of the bead chain links are broken, with the result that after pepsin has acted the bead chains instead of being 400 beads long are reduced to perhaps 20 or 40 bead lengths. Other enzymes from the intestinal tissue and from the pancreas gland are capable of reducing the protein to single beads. It takes many enzymes, however, to digest a protein completely. Each enzyme must have embroidered into its structure the right kind of pattern so it can hasten the breaking of a particular type of linkage between beads.

Two facts regarding enzymes stand out: first, they are produced within our bodies and are *not* necessary food ingredients; second, they are catalysts which hasten thousands of different reactions that take place in all our cells; digestion is only a small fraction of what they do.

In spite of their diverse activities enzymes are always proteins and can themselves, under appropriate conditions, be denatured and digested to yield the same beads that other proteins do. If they have other building units in their make-up as is often the case, they yield these too on being digested. We can and do eat "foreign" enzymes (e.g. from other organisms) but in general they are, as such, of no nutritional value, except as proteins. There should be no concern whether enzymes in foods (phosphatase in milk, for example) are destroyed during pasteurization or cooking since the bead chains need to be uncoiled and unraveled before they can be utilized as food.

Enzymes in our digestive juices and in all the cells of our body need to have their "native" characteristics in order to be active as catalysts. If the bead chain which enters into their structure is even partially uncoiled or unwound, the enzyme as such ceases to exist. It cannot now catalyze or hasten the reaction for which its original structure fitted it.

What does an enzyme do and how does it work? When we say it hastens a particular chemical reaction, we do not mean that it *forces* a reaction in a particular direction.

Most chemical reactions are reversible in nature. We sometimes represent a simple chemical reaction in which only two substances are involved as follows:

$$A \underset{\longleftarrow}{\overrightarrow{\hspace{2cm}}} B$$

This means that A can change into B, but that B can also change, at a lesser rate (as designated by the smaller arrow) into A. This designation does not tell us at all how rapidly the events take place. The interconversion may come to an equilibrium within a fraction of a second or it may take millions of years.

A catalyst, which an enzyme is, hastens the attainment of the equilibrium (balance) in reactions which otherwise would be slow. As one of my colleagues used to say, "A catalyst 'lubricates the arrows.'" It does not contribute any energy or driving force and functions essentially as a lubricant by making a reaction easy and fast. Like a lubricant it is not used up as a fuel is. It functions by its presence and is used over and over again.

Hydrogen gas and oxygen gas can be mixed together and, unless ignited by a spark, will remain an inert mixture of gases indefinitely. If we lead a mixture of these gases over palladium catalyst, they will combine to form water, and energy will be released. A small amount of palladium catalyst will cause the combination of a large amount of oxygen and hydrogen because the same palladium is used over and over. It furnishes no energy; it merely "lubricates" the reaction.

How does an enzyme act as a lubricant for a chemical reaction? An enzyme, which being a protein must be made up of relatively big molecules, must be built exactly right so that there is exact "sitting room" for the molecules it is going to affect. Each kind of molecule has a distinctive size and shape and the spot on the enzyme structure for a specific kind of molecule to attach must be "made to order" for that molecule. If the enzyme is to cause two different kinds of molecules to react (this is very common), the enzyme must have places for the two kinds to sit side by side for an instant of attachment. Because of their proximity and mode of attachment, the two molecules immediately interact. Once this happens the altered molecules lose their sitting places because they no longer fit; they cut loose and make room for another two molecules which then repeat the process. One large enzyme molecule can thus influence a very large number of reacting molecules in a twinkling of an eye, and chemical changes are brought about which in the practical sense wouldn't take place at all if the enzyme had not been present.

Each enzyme, and there are thousands of kinds, must be built in a distinctive way so it can catalyze one specific type of reaction. At all times reactions in great number are being catalyzed in this way in all the cells of our bodies. In living cells, enzymes are organized in such a way that the processes characteristic of that cell take place in an orderly fashion. Some processes, like the oxidation of food to obtain energy, which are taking place every second we live, involve many steps and many enzymes. Often the processes seem roundabout but there are reasons back of the operation. All the complex associations of structures and enzymes we sometimes call the metabolic machinery. Metabolism is everything that happens chemically within our bodies.

We have been discussing the chemical nature and the functioning of proteins and enzymes in nutrition. Proteins are valuable nutritionally because of the beads (the amino acids) they yield. Enzymes taken in the food are usually valuable for the same reason, and for this reason only. This does not mean that enzymes cannot be used medicinally but it does mean that food faddists who talk about the potent significance of the enzymes we eat are ill-informed. Sometimes they refer to "live" and "dead" enzymes. Since enzymes are protein molecules, they do not possess life, and hence can't be deprived of life. They can be denatured, of course, but this is a necessary step in their utilization as food. Enzymes as such are of little or no significance as constituents of foods. We make our own.

Other body constituents that originate within our bodies and are not usually obtained from food are the *hormones*. These vary greatly in chemical make-up; some are proteins and many are not. Their mode of action is poorly understood but they too must influence chemical reactions indirectly if not directly. Insulin with 51 beads is an example of a protein hormone; some hormones are similar to proteins in structure but are not classified as proteins because the molecules are too small (sometimes only 8 beads long). Other protein hormones may have 200 or more beads.

Some hormones are "steroids" and are more fatlike in their solubility; others are relatively simple nitrogen-containing molecules. From the nutritional standpoint hormones are *un*important, since while we often consume some of them, typically we make our own and do not depend upon any food source.

One hormone (that from the thyroid glands), has in its make-up an amino acid bead of unusual structure which contains iodine. When this hormone is consumed, this unique bead is made available so that consuming this hormone is effective. People who have, for surgical or other reasons, too little thyroid hormone can supplement their supply by taking thyroid tissue obtained from slaughtered animals and prepared for medicinal use. Other hormones, in some cases, are administered medicinally by mouth but, in general, hormones are insignificant constituents of foods. If the hormones consumed are protein in nature their bead chains are uncoiled and unwound and the beads broken apart during digestion to produce essentially the same products as those which other proteins yield. Such hormones when administered medicinally are given by injection in order to bypass the digestive system.

From this discussion it becomes apparent that nutritious food may contain thousands of proteins, but that they yield only twenty or so amino acids. All in all, however, nourishing food is an exceedingly complex mixture containing many different kinds of molecules.

It would be a hopeless situation if a layman had to scrutinize every bite and have it analyzed before he ate it. In the next chapter we will discuss important facts that have a direct bearing on the practical problem of how we can get what our bodies need.

IV

The Unity of Nature—
A Boon to Good Nutrition

Nature does not leave us in the predicament of having to analyze our diets for dozens of items before we know they are suitable to eat. If this restriction applied, if life were that complicated, the human race would not now be in existence. We avoid this necessity by consuming what nature has provided for us—from other organisms which resemble us in chemical make-up.

Why do we need such complex food as we do? Fundamentally the answer is this: Our bodies are complex chemical factories, deriving energy by carrying out a multitude of highly complicated chemical transformations, and the complex food that we eat is essential for the building and maintenance of this elaborate metabolic machinery.

The enzymes described in the previous chapter are integral and indispensable parts of the metabolic machinery of every kind of living thing. All living organisms from tiny bacteria to mammoth whales, from grasshoppers to giant sequoias are "in the same boat" in that they carry out their chemical transformations and derive their energy through the use of enzymes which they build within their cells. Furthermore, enzymes from all sources have *strong* resemblances. They are all protein in nature and are built from the very same kinds of beads. In addition, however, regardless of source, they often contain or require for their functioning one or more specific minerals such as calcium, magnesium, phosphate, iron, zinc, copper, cobalt, molybdenum, etc. They also frequently have in their make-up one or more of the vitamins such as vitamin B_1, niacinamide, riboflavin, pantothenic acid, pyridoxin or vitamin B_{12}. These occur practically universally in all organisms.

All organisms, regardless of type, must have the wherewithal to build these enzymes. Some organisms such as green plants have synthetic abilities far beyond what we human beings have. They can build their own beads and their own vitamins from simple chemicals but must depend on outside sources for the minerals.

We human beings, on the other hand, must obtain *in our food* not only numerous minerals but also the various vitamins and amino acids listed in capital letters on pages 21–23. We have the capability of building many complex chemical structures starting with these blocks, but the blocks themselves—all of them—must be furnished us in our food; otherwise we cannot by any means build our metabolic machinery.

The unity of nature is crucial for all life as we have it on earth. When a robin brings a worm or insect to feed its young, nature is providing a food that contains proteins which yield the very amino acids the young robin needs; also the same vitamins and minerals. If the worm or insect contained proteins built from amino acids foreign to the young robin's body, the young robin would be poisoned by them. If the vitamins were of a different variety, they would not nourish the young robin. If the minerals were unlike those used by the robin, they would be either useless or poisonous depending upon the amounts present.

There is, of course, among the millions of kinds of living things tremendous diversity along with astounding unity. Different organisms have different assortments of enzymes and carry out quite different processes. It is a fact, however, that of the 37 items listed as essential items in our diet, practically every one will be found in detectable amounts in *any* and *every* living organism. Living organisms from the simplest to the most complex types contain the same amino acids (*not* the same proteins), the same vitamins and the same minerals. Each enzyme has a distinctive make-up, but they all can be built from a relatively few units. The units are universal; the specific enzymes are different for every kind of organism.

In recent years, we hear of growing algae en route to feed spacemen during their prolonged journeys in space. This from the nutritional standpoint is not as preposterous as it may seem because algae build their enzymes and other cell constituents from the ground up, but when the cells are built, they contain essentially the same building blocks that we use. Algae can probably serve as a basic human food for this very reason. How good nutrition will be in such a case is still an open question.

A simple rule that will enable us down-to-earth people to get some of everything we need is this: Take a bite of some living organism! Plants usually do not bite back and hence are easy victims. Animals will serve too, but in this case it is safer—and less messy—to execute them first and eat them later.

Lest we take this rule too literally—it is good as far as it goes—we need to remind ourselves of the *quantitative aspects of nutrition* that we have asserted to be of paramount importance. It is not enough "to get some of everything we need." Every type of organism contains the vital items in proportions suitable for *its* needs. We need the same items in quantities suitable for *our* needs. If a person gets only half enough, in the case of one item only, he will be malnourished.

One amendment to the simple rule will improve our chances of getting a well-rounded diet. It is this: Don't restrict yourself to *one part* of a living organism, try to get the "whole works"! In the plant realm, do not restrict yourself to green leaves (spinach), or to roots (parsnips), or to seeds (corn or wheat), or to fruit (apples, tomatoes). Each of these is in itself incomplete. A combination diet containing leaves, roots, tubers, seeds, and fruits is a vast improvement. Early in the history of animal nutrition it was found that seeds and leaves have a profound supplementary action. Horses can live on oats, but if you wish to improve their nutrition materially give them grass or hay as well. Leaves in general contain minerals, for example, that supplement those in seeds.

In human nutrition the same principle holds whether one is considering plant food or animal food. A lack of appreciation of this principle appears in the all too common tendency to eat exclusively the *muscle* of slaughtered animals and to reject everything else. It is true that muscle tissue is the most abundant tissue and that eating the muscle of other animals should furnish us with food that will probably make continued existence possible. But this is not enough. We will get much better rounded nutrition (assuming we consume animal food exclusively) if we include in our diet some connective tissue, liver, glandular organs, sweetbreads, brains, skin, fat, and even gastrointestinal tissue (tripe).

There are those who for religious or other reasons abstain from animal food. Vegetarians can be well nourished if they eat wisely and include leaves, seeds, roots, and fruits in their diet. For the majority of Americans however, a mixed, diversified diet made up of both plant and animal foods seems most appropriate.

Before we leave the subject of how the unity of nature makes it vastly easier for us to select food that will maintain our lives, let us call attention to two relatively complete foods: *milk* (and dairy products generally) and eggs.

As is well known, milk is a relatively perfect food for young animals including young children. It is not quite perfect for an indefinite period—it lacks iron for one thing—but it has many virtues. Nature has prepared it for us; unlike most foods it is not one-sided, and the nutrition of most people would be improved if they consumed more of it. Cheeses and other dairy products have many of the advantages possessed by milk itself.

Eggs are valuable as a relatively complete food, because each egg has in it *everything* that is required to build a complete baby chick. Eggs contain all the building materials necessary for the nourishment of every kind of cell that enters into the make-up of an entire fowl, and for this reason constitute one of the most complete foods available. It is far from my purpose to urge the eating of eggs and more eggs. I merely call attention to their peculiar position as a well-rounded food. We will discuss in a later chapter, more specific suggestions as to how an individual may select his diet.

The extreme diversity that exists in nature, along with the remarkable unity, is worth a further look. Every kind of organism has its own inheritance—a complicated array of *genes* that are passed from one cell to its progeny. These genes have in their make-up an entirely different type of bead work from that present in the typical proteins. These beads contain phosphate as one distinguishing feature. Biochemists often call the gene bead work DNA's (deoxyribonucleic acids). The number of different kinds of genes existing in nature is almost infinitely large. The different DNA's resemble each other in the building blocks they contain; they differ in the internal arrangement of the blocks. In each of our fully constituted body cells we have at least hundreds of thousands of different genes.

These self-duplicating genes that were present in the original egg cells from which each of us developed, determine, among other things, our potentialities for building enzymes and other features of our metabolic machinery.

If a rat has metabolic machinery different from that of a guinea pig, this is because the different animals have different sets of genes that control their potentialities for producing the enzymes and other structures. If we were compiling a "nutritional *must* list" for rats, we would end up with a list strongly resembling that compiled (in capital letters) for human beings (p. 21–23). However, the list of amino-acid beads would not be identical and we could leave vitamin C (ascorbic acid) off the list, because rats' genes furnish the potentialities for producing enzymes that can build ascorbic acid from simpler molecules. A nutritional *must* list for guinea pigs would be slightly different from that for human beings, but guinea pigs' genes, like human genes, carry no potential for building ascorbic acid. This vitamin is therefore an essential in the diets of both guinea pigs and humans.

The unity of nature is exhibited in the fact that the tissues of rats have a relative abundance of ascorbic acid in them. Rats use ascorbic acid in their metabolic machinery, but they can make their own.

Every kind of organism has its own type of gene assortment; each kind therefore has its own nutritional requirements. Most mammals have requirements that bear many resemblances to each other, though there are some striking differences such as those we have noted.

Not only are there differences between the gene assortments in different species of animals; each individual animal has a distinctive assortment which causes different individual animals to build the various enzymes with unequal ease. This fact is particularly important for human beings, each of whom has somewhat unique metabolic machinery due to differing gene assortments. This is one place where the quantitative aspects of nutrition come into play. Human gene assortments are characteristic of human beings and cause us to have need for nutrients in *amounts* that are suitable for us but not most suitable for some other species. Likewise each individual person with a unique gene assortment has need for nutrients in *amounts* that are most suitable for him or her but not so suitable for another individual whose gene assortment and metabolic machinery are different. That individual people have different and distinctive metabolic machineries is strikingly evidenced by the well-known fact that bloodhounds (for example) can distinguish people by the odors of their metabolic products. They could not do this if our metabolisms were all the same.

The unity of nature helps us tremendously in choosing our food wisely, but wise choices do not come automatically. Later in this book we will discuss other helps that nature gives us. We had better take nature's help when it is offered.

Nature has revealed to us her unity, and with it the assurance that if we nourish ourselves with a diversified selection of foods derived from living organisms, we are most likely to nourish ourselves well. This use of nature must be intelligent. No one can be intelligent about nutritional matters unless he has some substantial training in biochemistry because enzymes, vitamins, amino acids, minerals, etc., are all chemicals. Uninformed spokesmen espousing the cause of "nature" (including sometimes physicians with poor training) sometimes refer to "living" and "dead" vitamins and to *killing* vitamins and enzymes. All vitamins and enzymes are chemical substances; they are never endowed with life and hence cannot be killed.

The unity of nature has existed for millions of years. Long before men appeared on the earthly scene there were the same amino acids, vitamins, and minerals as we have today. Every evidence indicates that throughout geological time, these basic ingredients have played an indispensable role in the life of living things. If we try to fight this unity or forget its existence, our efforts are likely to be futile.

V

What Types of Ills May Be
Due to Faulty Nutrition?

If an academic student of nutrition were asked in a university or civil service examination "What diseases are due to nutritional deficiency?" he would probably be expected to answer: rickets, scurvy, beriberi, pellagra, night blindness, and kwashiorkor. Many physicians, reflecting what they have been taught in medical schools, might answer the question in about the same way with a few amplifications.

This answer, based on concepts which are now passé in informed biochemical circles, is pitifully inadequate and incomprehensive. Cellular malnutrition, which is the basis of all malnutrition, is probably at the roots of ten times as many disease conditions as the clinically defined deficiency diseases listed above.

Since every cell and tissue in our bodies needs nourishment, and each part may be subjected to nutrition which is faulty in varying degrees, the number of human ills that may arise because of imperfect nutrition is very large. Faulty cellular nutrition of one type or another may be a basic cause of most of the noninfective diseases—diseases that are at present poorly controlled by medical science.

It is one of the tasks of nutritional biochemistry and medicine in the future to determine how many of these uncontrolled metabolic diseases are caused by cellular malnutrition, and how they can be brought under control.

Let us consider first, diseases or deficiencies associated with reproduction. Obviously, it would be impractical to carry out experiments with human beings, designed to find out how reproductive capacity is affected by diet. Such experiments have, however, been carried out using various experimental animals. Reproductive failure can be brought about by a large number of different deficiencies.

We have already mentioned that rats lacking enough vitamin A or enough vitamin E fail to reproduce. Lack of enough manganese causes male rats to lose their mating interest and, if prolonged, causes them to be sterile. Lack of sufficient highly unsaturated fat acids (linoleic acid) causes sterility, as do lacks involving any one of the amino acids essential for rats.

In a very real sense, every item on the must list for rats (it is very similar to but not identical with the human must list on pages 21–23) is necessary for their fertility because, without *all of them*, no animal can be raised to the point where it can mate and reproduce.

It is for reasons based upon this discussion that the term "the antisterility vitamin" which has sometimes been used to designate vitamin E, is unwarranted. Such a designation is based upon a most limited appreciation of the facts as they are now known. The B vitamins, for example, are all in a real sense antisterility vitamins. The essential amino acids and minerals are also antisterility nutrients.

Physicians and others are entirely justified in their rejection of the idea that vitamin E is a cure for human sterility or that human sterility necessarily has its roots in vitamin E deficiency. Different species of mammals respond differently to specific nutritional lacks. Present knowledge does permit the strong suggestion that cellular malnutrition is probably a highly important factor in human infertility, but knowledge has not advanced far enough so that we can say that any one lack—vitamin A, manganese, vitamin E, highly unsaturated fat acids, one of the essential amino acids, or one of the B vitamins—is most important. It is probable that in different cases of sterility, different lacks are involved. This is a field for future research.

Inborn deformities in human beings may have malnutrition as a basis. This is evidenced by the fact that deformities in great variety have been produced in experimental animals (pigs, rabbits, rats, mice) by inducing one or another nutritional deficiency in the pregnant females.

Vitamin A deficiency, riboflavin deficiency, folic acid deficiency, vitamin B_{12} deficiency, pantothenic acid deficiency, and vitamin E deficiency have all yielded striking structural abnormalities. Among the defects observed are: small eyes, lack of eyes, deformed eyes, eyes open at birth (rats), brain malformations, heart malformations, displaced heart, aorta defects, kidney defects, hermaphroditism, genito-urinary abnormalities, shortening or absence of foot and leg bones or of jaw bones, cleft palate, harelip, absence of toes, extra toes, open abdomen, closed esophagus, hernia of the diaphragm.

It is interesting that in several instances a deficiency at *a particular time* during the gestation period may cause abnormalities but later on the same deficiency may be relatively ineffective. This emphasizes the importance of completely adequate nutrition during the stage when organs and structures are first being formed.

Human experiments designed to find out whether specific deficiencies will produce deformed babies are unthinkable, but experimental attempts to improve human diets to see if they will bring about improved reproduction have been carried out, for example, in Oslo, Norway by Guttorm Toverud. In this 5–6-year study, attempted improvement of the nutrition of mothers caused stillbirths to be cut down to about half. Premature births were diminished more than 50 per cent, mortality of infants within the first month and within the first year were each decreased almost as much, while rickets and other evidence of bone deficiency as well as brain hemorrhage practically disappeared.

Many ailments of the prospective mothers which are common during pregnancy such as anemia, cramps in legs, numbness of fingers and toes, neuralgic pains, constipation, raised blood pressure, and edema were also greatly benefited by the improved nutrition, as was also the breast-feeding ability of the mothers after their babies were born.

Such results are impressive because, in a large-scale study such as this, the attempted nutritional improvement could only have been successful to a modest degree. The eating habits and behavior of people cannot be controlled in the same way that those of experimental animals in cages can.

An interesting problem has to do with the effect of nutrition on infective diseases. Early in this century it was found that experimental animals made deficient in vitamin A were far more subject to various infections of the eyes and of the respiratory tract. Some enthusiasts were inclined to label vitamin A the "antiinfective vitamin." Such a designation was rightly resisted by members of the medical profession and public health authorities. Since that time numerous observations have implicated other vitamins in resistance to infection. Vitamin C, for example, seems to play an important role in "antibody" formation and on this basis may be regarded as antiinfective.

The truth is, of course, that every amino acid, mineral, and vitamin which contributes to the health and vigor of one's body is in a sense an antiinfective agent, because resistance to disease is a *sine qua non* of continued existence, and resistance is the highest in those in which the cells and tissues most intimately involved in disease-resistance processes, are nourished at the highest level of excellence.

Several studies have indicated that improved nutrition helps in the control of tuberculosis. One of these studies took place in a hospital where the patients were already characterized as "exceedingly well nourished" by an outside physician. The patients were secretly divided into two groups: one group received nutritional supplements, the other group received similar-appearing supplements that were devoid of any food value. None of the attendants or patients knew which individuals were getting the real thing and which were getting "blanks."

As a result of this experiment it was found, after totaling up the reports on all the patients, that those getting the nutritional supplements were better off in many respects—improvement in chest X rays, rapidity of discharge as cured, healthiness of appetites, weight gains (almost twice as large), decreased restlessness and desire for continual attention. While the general role of nutrition in favoring the recovery of tuberculosis patients has long been recognized and no tuberculosis hospital worthy of the name would consciously neglect the nutrition of the patients, it becomes apparent from this study that being "exceedingly well nourished" in the medically accepted sense is not enough for tuberculosis patients.

Whether the particular nutritional supplements used in this hospital study were the very best possible, can seriously be debated. This is not as important as the finding that the supplements used actually brought marked benefit to a group which by ordinary standards was already very well nourished.

Diseases of the digestive tract may have, in some cases at least, a nutritional basis. One of the early observations made on pantothenic acid, the vitamin with which I worked for many years, was that when pigs were given a diet deficient in it, the entire lining of the digestive tract from one end to the other was spotted with many ulcers. Can we deduce from this fact that whenever pigs, human or porcine, get stomach or duodenal ulcers, it must be due to pantothenate deficiency? Obviously not. Ulcers are in essence "sores" and sores may have many causes.

When one develops a duodenal ulcer while consuming no harmful food or damaging chemicals, this suggests that the ulcer has an internal origin (that is, within the duodenal tissue); if so, nutritional inadequacy suggests itself and the fact that ulcers can definitely be produced in animals by nutritional lack is worth considering. The idea that nutrition plays a role in the production of human duodenal ulcers is indicated by the work of my colleague, Dr. William Shive, who, collaborating with a group of physicians, has found in an extensive well-controlled study that ulcers heal more rapidly when glutamine (one of the nutritional substances listed in italics on page 21) is administered to the patients.

Two opposing ailments involving the digestive tract—diarrhea and constipation—are often, under different conditions, the results of faulty nutrition. If, however, all the nerve and muscle cells associated with the intestinal tract are well nourished and healthy, the motility in the tract is held at a desirable level—the intestinal contents are neither stagnated nor are they pushed along so rapidly that absorption is almost nil. One nutritional factor that is known to be concerned in this process (by inference, *all* nutritional factors are concerned) is the vitamin pantothenic acid, already mentioned. Often after the stress of an operation, patients are in great pain and difficulty because the intestinal muscles become in effect paralyzed; movements virtually cease, gas accumulates and severe abdominal pain results. It has been found in this condition (paralytic ileus) that the administration of suitable doses of pantothenate often causes intestinal movements to start, the gas is expelled and the normal functioning of the intestine is restored. Since pantothenate is a completely bland innocuous substance without any irritating or pharmacological action whatever, the question arises: How does it act? The only remotely reasonable answer is that it acts *nutritionally* to bring back health to the stressed and deficient intestinal tissues. Only by being built into enzyme systems within cells does pantothenate have any effect.

It seems highly probable that if the cells and tissues of the gastrointestinal tract are continuously well nourished, many digestive and related ailments will disappear. Conversely, many such ailments can be produced by malnutrition. It has been observed many times that some individuals appear to suffer from a particular deficiency even though plenty of the nutrient in question may be in their food. *Absorption* may be the weak link in the chain. Recently it has been observed, for example, that the vitamin A in the diet may be incompletely absorbed, but that when vitamin E is furnished in abundance, vitamin A is readily absorbed and deficiency of vitamin A disappears.

Diseases of the circulatory system can have as their basis nutritional insufficiency. One of the most interesting of these is anemia. The blood carries enormous numbers of red cells (about 5 billion per thimbleful) which have as their main constituent the oxygen-carrying, bright-red protein, hemoglobin. These red cells (corpuscles) are unusual as body cells go, because by the time they mature (in mammals) they have lost their nuclei and have no powers of reproduction. They persist in the body for a few weeks until they are "worn out" and have to be replaced with new ones. The production of these new replacement cells constitutes, in adults, an exacting task involving relatively extensive protein synthesis.

Anemia involves a deficiency of the number of these corpuscles or of their hemoglobin content. It has been produced experimentally in animals as a result of several specific nutritional deficiencies. Without sufficient iron, people or animals become anemic; this is understandable because hemoglobin contains iron as one of its basic ingredients. An insufficiency of any one of the essential amino acids may produce anemia and this is understandable because these building stones are part of the make-up of the protein itself. Anemia can also be produced, however, by limiting any one of a number of other nutrients—substances which do not occur as constituents of hemoglobin. Why can lack of copper, vitamin B_{12} (which contains cobalt) folic acid, niacin, pyridoxin or ascorbic acid —any *one* of these—produce anemia, when these are not constituents of hemoglobin? The answer is simply this: the living cells which give rise to the red cells need these other items in order that they can produce hemoglobin and the red cells that contain it. Anything that can cripple these living cells is capable of producing anemia. It is revealing that so many different individual lacks have actually been proved to produce this disease.

Another condition involving the circulatory system which has been repeatedly observed in connection with nutritional lacks is *edema*. In this condition there is a failure of the regulatory mechanisms which control the water balance in the body and as a result tissues become puffy and overloaded with water. In so-called *"wet"* beriberi is an example of edema produced because of a nutritional lack of vitamin B_1 (and perhaps other essentials as well). Edema has been observed to result from amino-acid deficiencies, from deficiencies of B vitamins, from lack of unsaturated fat acids, and from general starvation. Control of water balance involves the functioning of living cells and an upset of this balance is one of the common signs of malnutrition.

A specific lack (vitamin K) is known to lessen the coagulation power of the blood. This ability to coagulate is a most vital protective mechanism which prevents people from bleeding to death every time their skin is scratched. The coagulation of the blood is a highly complicated process and vitamin K is only one factor. It is worthy of note, however, that normal coagulation can be abolished by a nutritional lack.

High blood pressure—lack of control of blood pressure—is another difficulty which in humans *may have* a nutritional origin. The most conclusive studies on this have been done with experimental animals. A series of 36 well-nourished control rats had blood pressures of 118 (average of systolic and diastolic). Rats raised in the same way except that they were made deficient for 5 or 6 days in early life in the essential choline (page 22) but were well nourished the rest of their lives, had comparable blood pressures of 165, and up to as high as 230. Animals made deficient in choline for a few days during their youth suffered kidney damage—mild to severe— and the heart size was made to increase in proportion to the kidney damage and the increased blood pressure. Thus there was observed a whole series of changes involving the heart, kidneys, and blood pressure—all the result of depriving young animals during youth *for only a few days* of one essential nutrient.

There are dangers in attempting to draw conclusions applicable to human beings, from such an experiment with rats. One danger involves centering one's attention on choline, as *the thing* to watch in connection with heart, kidney, and blood-pressure difficulties. Rats may have peculiarities in this regard which human beings do not show. Another dangerous conclusion would be that all heart enlargement, kidney damage, or high blood pressure must of necessity be the result of choline or other nutritional deficiencies. The fact that rats can suffer from all of these difficulties *as a direct result of nutritional deficiency* should put us on our guard, however, and make us wonder whether comparable human difficulties may not be caused by nutritional lacks. If these changes can be brought about in rats by nutritional deficiency, they may also appear in humans as a result of imperfect cellular nutrition.

Recent studies by Harvard investigators have revealed the occurrence of kidney stones in experimental animals and the prevention of their occurrence by adequate amounts of magnesium and pyridoxin. It thus becomes probable that in human beings such ailments may have faulty nutrition as their basis.

Too much salt in the diet may contribute to the production of high blood pressure and the use of low-salt diets have been widely recommended in this connection. Sometimes they are called "salt-free diets" which is not strictly correct, since foods in general contain salt even if none is added. Salt is one of the essentials without which we cannot live. Recently, evidence has been obtained at the Brookhaven National Laboratory that incompletely purified salt from ocean water contains impurities which induce high blood pressure, and that pure sodium chloride is less effective. If this is confirmed it will put a question mark after the idea often expressed that sea salt (not highly purified) is superior to the purified chemical.

We have already mentioned the fact that dogs made deficient in pantothenic acid died suddenly with heart as well as other involvements. Human-heart difficulties of many sorts are associated with nutritional deficiencies. In beriberi which involves primarily a vitamin B_1 deficiency, heart damage always appears sooner or later and death comes as a result of heart failure.

Again we must be on our guard against jumping to hasty conclusions. We must not indulge ourselves in the belief that all heart failures have a nutritional origin because some of them definitely do. Failure of the heart, like that of any organ, however, *may have* a nutritional basis, and it is unsafe to overlook this origin as a possibility.

In this connection it will be well to discuss more fully the most common type of heart failure—coronary heart disease— which kills nearly a half million people annually in the United States. This disease is related to nutrition, though somewhat indirectly. Fundamentally, in an acute attack the heart muscle fails for a lack of oxygen which is normally carried to it through the coronary artery in the oxygenated blood. When the coronary artery is partially or completely stopped up, the oxygenated blood cannot get through adequately.

The stoppage of the coronary artery is therefore the crucial event. This happens when the interior surface of this artery develops an unhealthy condition; the situation then becomes ripe for the continued deposition of jagged cholesterol crystals and for the formation of blood clots which tend (other things being equal) to form in the presence of rough surfaces. The unhealthy condition of the artery wall, the deposition of cholesterol, and the excessive tendency of the blood to clot may all be influenced by nutrition.

The complete story of nutrition and its relation to coronary heart disease cannot be told because there are still "unknowns." Cholesterol is associated with fats in food; some fats are relatively high in cholesterol, others are low. But the avoidance of excessive cholesterol in the food is certainly not of prime importance because cholesterol is produced in our bodies when we consume none whatever. The avoidance of cholesterol production in the body is a worthy objective for those who have an inborn susceptibility to coronary disease, and on the basis of present knowledge this can be best accomplished by reducing the fat intake without, however, eliminating the desirable unsaturated fats (p. 21). Most vegetable oils (except coconut oil) are relatively rich in unsaturated fats. Hydrogenated fats which are partially solidified by hydrogenation are inferior in this respect to the original oils from which they are made.

There are doubtless other causes that contribute to coronary heart disease. The use of tobacco by susceptible individuals probably contributes materially; one's whole mode of life particularly with respect to exercise is another factor. There is small doubt, however, even in our present state of ignorance that the kind of food one eats—its complete adequacy (not usually sufficiently stressed) and freedom from excessive saturated fats—is a tremendously important factor contributing to the continuing health of all the cells in our artery walls and both directly and indirectly to the health of the heart muscles themselves.

Strokes of apoplexy result from failure of brain cells to get the nourishment they need. Rupture of blood vessels (hemorrhage) or plugging of blood vessels by clots (thrombus formation) can bring this about. Good nutrition helps maintain healthy blood vessels which do not rupture easily, and also helps prevent the formation of plugs which stop blood flow. Recent studies have indicated that the administration of rutin and related glucosides (p. 22) may be a factor in preventing successive strokes after an individual has already had a slight one. The evidence on this point is not incontrovertible.

There are numerous metabolic diseases such as gout, diabetes, and obesity in which nutrition undoubtedly plays an important role, yet there are also predisposing factors which make particular individuals susceptible to them. An individual who has a tendency toward gout has a relatively high level of uric acid in the blood that may have its origin in foods or may be produced within the body itself. Inability of the kidneys to eliminate uric acid adequately may also be a factor. Nutrition may be involved in gout not only because certain foods may yield uric acid but also because excellent nutrition of all the cells and tissues involved (including kidney tissues) would be expected to promote the control of uric-acid production and disposal.

Diabetes is a complicated disease which involves an imbalance between insulin production (in the pancreas) and functional activities of the liver, adrenal glands, and the pituitary glands. Hundreds of studies have been made in the hope of better control of the disease by diet, but without a recognition of the other factors, control of diet is futile. Excessive carbohydrate consumption is contraindicated in diabetes; it is desirable that carbohydrates be produced within the body from proteins and certain other food constituents. A serious difficulty arises in the nourishment of diabetics because restrictions which may be instituted may cause them to become deficient in ways that are not anticipated. A diabetic individual, like anyone else, needs a completely adequate diet so that his pancreas, liver, adrenals, and pituitary (as well as other tissues) are fully nourished. Though the connection between diabetes and nutrition involves many unknowns, it is entirely reasonable to suppose that excellent nutrition will prevent—if anything will—the development of diabetes in those who in earlier life do not have the disease.

Obesity has nutritional roots because it cannot take place unless unburned food accumulates. There are probably several types of obesity and gradations between them. For example, there is evidence that in some cases fat accumulates because of a metabolic imbalance which involves greediness on the part of the fat cells; they tend to rob the other tissues, with the result that the individual may be malnourished in many respects while the fat cells pile up unnecessary reserves. If the individual eats less to correct the overweight, the other cells and tissues of the body may suffer and the fat cells do not bear the brunt of the deprivation.

An important factor in many cases of obesity is a lack of balance between appetite and bodily needs. When this balance is disturbed in the direction of surplus food consumption and assimilation, by any cause whatever, obesity results. The disturbance need be only very slight. A healthy individual may consume as much as 8 tons of moist food in the course of ten years. If only 99.5 per cent of this food (instead of 100 per cent) is burned up or rejected as waste, this would mean a weight gain of 80 pounds! This lack of balance may be contributed to by emotional and psychological factors—our thoughts and emotions do affect our body chemistry—and hormonal influences also doubtless come into play.

Sometimes one reads the statement that Americans are not *mal*nourished, rather they tend to be *over*nourished. This,

in one sense, is true; yet there is quite a different way of looking at the problem. The appestat which regulates the quantity
of food that is eaten must have a cellular basis; the indications
are that the primary mechanism is located in the hypothalamus of the brain. These nerve cells require nourishment and
it is possible—indeed highly probable, in my opinion—that
obesity is often *a disease of deficient nutrition*, that is, poor
nutrition of the nervous tissues involved in the control of
food consumption. It is possible that this poor nutrition dates
back to early childhood (or earlier) and that individuals who
tend strongly to be obese have had their appetite mechanism more or less permanently deranged by bad nutrition.
There is hope, however, when the story of nutrition is more
fully known, that the deficient nutrition of those who have
a strong tendency to be obese can be corrected to such an
extent that weight control is as easy and automatic as it is
with many other more fortunate members of the human
family.

One of the bases for this hope lies in the fact that nutritional deficiencies do cause anorexia (lack of appetite), which
is one direction in which the appetite mechanism can fail.
Hyperorexia (excessive appetite) likewise has a physiological
basis. There is no doubt whatever that there is a nervous
mechanism in the body which controls food consumption.
The cells and tissues involved are capable of being nourished
at various levels of efficiency. When these cells and tissues are
perfectly well, the individual is able to rely on this "governor"
implicitly year after year and decade after decade without any
difficulty whatever. Millions of people, especially when they
do not shun exercise, have lived their entire lives without
ever having had at any time a weight problem. Such individuals eat exactly the right amount, automatically.

The author has accumulated a large amount of information
that indicates alcoholic craving (an appetite derangement)
has its origin in the deficient nutrition of the cells in the nerv-

ous tissues involved, but this is too large a subject to discuss at this point. Everyone agrees that excessive alcohol consumption makes for malnutrition and that cirrhosis of the liver, for example, is caused by vital nutritional lacks.

The bearing of nutrition on arthritic and rheumatic diseases is obscure because the origin and causes of these diseases are largely unknown. Various vitamins have been implicated at different times, but in general the reported connection between such deficiencies and these diseases has not been confirmed. It is notable that anyone prescribing diets for arthritic or rheumatic individuals is likely to emphasize the importance of a well-rounded diet containing an abundance of proteins, minerals, and vitamins.

A practicing physician, Dr. William Kaufman, in Connecticut, has made a very extended study of diseases of the joints and has found stiffening of the joints to be relieved in most individuals by the use of niacinamide, one of the B vitamins. He has sought to get highly quantitative results by careful measurement of the flexing of the various joints in the body of an individual before and during the course of treatment. From the complicated data of the various angles of flexion he obtains a composite "joint-range index" for any given individual at any time. In young children this index approaches 100 but progressively decreases with age so that in a group of untreated patients it averaged in the 60's for those over 55 years of age.

When these patients were given relatively massive doses of niacinamide for a period of months, the joint-range index (*presumably* an objective determination) increased from 87.4 to 95.9 in six children in the 6–10 age group; from 78 to 88.3 in 31 individuals in the 26–30 age group; from 70.3 to 83.8 in 41 individuals in the 51–55 age group; and from 61.5 to 77.9 in 16 individuals in the 65–70 age group.

These results appear to be clear cut and, unless one wishes to entertain ideas of deliberate misrepresentation or of gross self-delusion, they should be taken seriously and investigated further. Clinical facilities for checking such results as these (such a study would cost a tidy sum) are most often lacking, and practicing physicians must in general either accept or reject them as they stand. Since these findings do not fit in well with ideas that are currently in fashion they are most often ignored.

One of the factors which makes the study of arthritic and rheumatic diseases difficult is the existence of individual susceptibility. It seems most probable that many nutritional and other factors are involved in such diseases and that what applies to one susceptible individual may not apply to another.

One is led to wonder in connection with the observations of Dr. Kaufman why such large doses of niacinamide are necessary when human bodies are usually satisfied with amounts perhaps $\frac{1}{10}$ of that which he prescribed. In attempting to understand this problem one needs to bear in mind that joints involve living cells which require nourishment. It is possible that for some reason not at present recognized, the crucial cells in an arthritic individual do not get the niacinamide they need unless the blood and tissues are highly loaded with an excess.

One of the reasons for mentioning the pioneering work of Dr. Kaufman is because his findings are in line with a broad principle which no intelligent student of arthritis can fail to recognize—namely that to function properly, joints like any other part of the body require continuous good nutrition. This physician claims to have found an important missing link. It would be absurd to think that joints require niacinamide and nothing else. It is too much to hope that niacinamide is a completely effective specific cure for all types of arthritic disease. It is not too much to hope, however, that when the story of nutrition unfolds more completely, a way will be found to nourish joints effectively, so that gross abnormalities of function can be eliminated.

In this connection it will be well to discuss briefly the problem of aging as it is related to nutrition. One of the most consistent symptoms of aging is the progressive stiffening of one's joints. If this does not take place too prematurely, it must be accepted and lived with. According to the fundamental ideas on which this little book is based, good nutrition should be an important factor in delaying the aging process. Different parts of the body age at different rates—every student of geriatrics accepts this as a fact—so that each individual as he ages may remain relatively young in some respects while becoming relatively old in others. We are not built like Oliver Wendell Holmes' "Wonderful One Hoss Shay" which retained its complete faculties unimpaired until the dramatic moment when it instantly completely disintegrated.

It would seem desirable on the basis of common sense for each of us as we age to favor our weakest member with the best possible nutrition for the cells and tissues involved in it. If we have a tendency toward arthritis (which in some cases may be merely a premature aging of the joints), then it would seem sensible to furnish our joints with abundance of the particular nutrients for which the joints are likely to have special need. If an individual's kidneys, or colon, or adrenals, or heart, etc., is aging prematurely, then it should have special attention, if possible. I predict that physicians in the future will become expert in diagnosing each individual's aging processes, and in suggesting to each individual how he can best nourish his aging body. For the present, nothing can take the place of a well-rounded nutritional supply of everything that our body's cells and tissues need.

There are many diseases of the organs and tissues where the special senses reside—eyes, ears, nose, tongue, and skin —that have a nutritional basis.

The discovery of vitamin A centered around an eye disease called xerophthalmia which was produced in rats when vitamin A was lacking in the diet. Its lack, besides impairing vision, also affected epithelial tissue so that it became unhealthy, failed to secrete mucus and to protect itself from outside infection. This can happen around the eyes as well as in the respiratory tract and in many other parts of the body. Subsequently, it has become established that vitamin A is absolutely essential to vision in man and all animals and its deficiency causes various degrees of night blindness and snow blindness in humans. I had a partially color-blind student who carefully studied himself and found repeatedly that his color vision improved when he took relatively large doses of vitamin A and deteriorated again when he ceased using this supplement.

Riboflavin (vitamin B_2) deficiency is also known to produce cataracts in the eyes of a large number of experimental animals. If the deficiency is not too prolonged the cataracts disappear when riboflavin is supplied. Human cataracts have in specific cases also been benefited by the administration of generous amounts of riboflavin. Again, one should not hastily conclude that cataracts are always the result of riboflavin deficiency. Actually, cataracts have been caused in experimental animals by making them deficient in some of the essential amino acids, and vitamin C deficiency has also been implicated in both animal and human cataracts. It is reasonable to suppose that any one of several nutritional deficiencies may be basic to the formation of cataracts. Nor does this, of course, exclude other possible causative factors.

While difficulties of hearing are not usually associated with nutritional deficiencies, the studies of Dr. Miles Atkinson of New York indicate that Ménière's syndrome which commonly exhibits itself by dizziness, progressive deafness, and distressing ringing of the ears, results from malnutrition. Many of his cases, including several different types, responded to relatively large doses of niacinamide, riboflavin, and thiamin, and in some cases the clearing up of the condition was remarkably satisfactory. Of course it was impossible to carry out strictly controlled experiments. Whether the results would have been far better if a more generous assortment of nutritional elements were used, remains to be seen; in any event he reported that a substantial percentage of his patients were greatly relieved by nutritional treatment. We thus have further evidence that certain portions of one's anatomy (the inner-ear structures, including nerves, in this case) may be malnourished to the point of serious impairment, while the rest of the body still functions reasonably satisfactorily.

One of the classic ways of diagnosing illness is to look at the patient's tongue. Gross deficiencies of B vitamins show up relatively consistently here and while it would lead us too far afield to discuss details, it is evident that the nervous structures involved in tasting as well as those in the nose and throat which are involved in flavor detection need continual nourishment. If this nourishment is inadequate many structural and functional impairments result. Physicians who are practiced in the art are able to gain much information about the patient's deficiencies by careful examination of his or her tongue. Clues as to deficiencies of riboflavin, niacin, pyridoxin, folic acid, pantothenic acid, and cobalamin (vitamin B_{12}) can be gathered by examination of the mouth and tongue. The teeth and gums are also capable of suffering from malnutrition in line with our previous discussion. Whether the mouth region is a perfect index of deficiencies in many other parts of the body is another question, and in my opinion a highly debatable one.

The skin is a region which is known to be affected by many nutritional lacks. Scarcely a deficiency exists which does not manifest itself by pathological changes in the skin. This has been demonstrated particularly in animals, where it is possible to carry out conclusive experiments. The number of reports of human diseased-skin conditions that are improved by supplying deficient nutrients is large, and we will not attempt to review these. Suffice it to say that there is evidence that acne, eczemas, dermatitis (a general term for skin inflammation), and even psoriasis (a condition which is almost, by definition, mysterious and incurable) may in specific cases have a nutritional origin. Acne usually involves infections, but well-nourished skin appears to be able to resist such infections. Eczemas and rashes may have many causes but they are often completely eliminated as a result of better nutrition. Reliable reports of cases in which conditions diagnosed as psoriasis have been eliminated by the use of nutritional supplements, have been published. Among the many nutrients that have been implicated in diseased conditions of the skin and hair are vitamin A, vitamin D, vitamin E, vitamin C, thiamin, riboflavin, pantothenic acid, biotin, vitamin B_6, unsaturated fat acids, inositol, para-aminobenzoic acid, and essential amino acids. Even this is not an exhaustive list.

The complications of allergies often enter into skin as well as other difficulties. Whenever one suffers from an allergic reaction, the body is put under stress. Fully adequate nutrition helps the body withstand stress and is an important defense against the difficulties that ensue. Emotional stresses and those arising from irradiation with X rays are also partially counteracted by high-quality nutrition.

Three other types of conditions: chilblains, the "burning-foot syndrome" and wound healing, all involving the skin and allied structures, are thought to be influenced by nutrition. Generally improved nutrition in children such as brought about by increasing their milk consumption is reported to decrease the incidence of chilblains; the burning-foot syndrome has been combated by administering pantothenate, and wound healing is said to be hastened by generous amounts of ascorbic acid—also by generally improved nutrition, including plenty of high-quality protein. One physician recommends from two to seven times the regular maintenance level of protein in order to promote the healing of bed sores.

The large list of diseases that is known to be influenced by nutrition includes those classed as nervous and mental diseases. These range from those in which definite nerve structures are known to be impaired, to those in which the nerve involvement is vague but none the less basic. They range from mild disorders which are not commonly regarded as "diseases" at all, up to the most severe mental diseases known.

Early in the history of vitamin research, fowls and birds fed exclusively on polished rice, and rats made deficient in what was then known as vitamin B developed polyneuritis, a diseased condition associated with loss of coordinated movement, and, in rats, the loss of the use of the hind legs. Nerves were proved by microscopic examination to be diseased and degenerated. The prominence of nerve symptoms in cases of lack of vitamin B_1, was responsible for the name "aneurin" used widely in Britain and European countries to designate vitamin B_1. The fallacy of saying "vitamin B_1 is for nerves" has already been pointed out. This fallacy is borne out by recognition of the fact that pantothenate deficiency and vitamin B_{12} deficiency, to cite two examples, both give rise to pathological nerves just as does the lack of vitamin B_1. If vitamin B_1 is an aneurin (a preventer of nervous disease) so are pantothenate and vitamin B_{12}, as well as (theoretically at least) many, many other nutrients.

One of the facts discovered early in vitamin research is that animals having insufficient vitamin B_1 lose their appetites. This must involve malnutrition of nerve cells because the regulation of appetite involves a nervous function. Pigeons were once a favorite animal used in vitamin B_1 research. If they were given an exclusive diet of polished rice and allowed to eat voluntarily, they would frequently die of starvation, because their appetite mechanism failed. Only when force-fed the polished rice would they live long enough to develop typical polyneuritis.

One of the first symptoms of vitamin B_1 deficiency as produced in human volunteers is the very same symptom—anorexia or loss of appetite. While it would be unsafe to conclude that whenever human beings lack appetite, there must be lack of vitamin B_1, yet it is a well-known fact that appetite can be turned off and on by this nutritional element, and it seems safe to conclude on the basis of all we know about appetites, that nutritional lacks of one kind or another are probably highly important causes of loss of appetite.

Lack of mental vigor, and lack of ability to concentrate, are other symptoms that have been shown in specific cases to be due to nutritional lacks. Controlled studies with school children both in this country and abroad have shown that when their nutrition is improved (often by giving them a larger supply of milk) their ability to work and play is markedly increased along with their alertness and mental vigor. Recently, the relation between mental vigor and good nutrition was observed in the Purdue University laboratories where volunteer students were observed in different levels of intake of the amino acid lysine (p. 21). With 500 milligrams per day, one subject (RBC) appeared to be getting along satisfactorily until he suddenly decided to withdraw from the experiment because he could not concentrate on his studies, was tired all the time, and was in danger of failing his forthcoming mid-semester examinations. His lysine supply was immediately increased to 1,500 milligrams daily. Within 48 hours his bodily retention of nitrogen increased; his mental vigor and feeling of well being returned and he voluntarily kept on the diet—with increased lysine—without difficulty or complaint.

The definite need for various essential amino acids (p. 21 –22) by human beings has been established, but not without specific experiments with individuals. Dr. William Rose, who was a pioneer in this field, noted that when young men were deprived of essential amino acids they sometimes became peevish, irritable, and hard to get along with, whereas these symptoms disappeared when the essential amino acids were returned in abundance to their diet. This observation coupled with the fact that when volunteer groups of conscientious objectors were placed on semistarvation diets during World War II, they often exhibited irritability and other forms of psychoneurosis as a result, leads us to suspect that nutritional inadequacies have more to do with symptoms of this kind than is commonly supposed. This suspicion is further confirmed by the fact that human vitamin B_1 deficiency, as demonstrated by direct experiment with volunteers, results in many cases in irritability, anxiety, increased sensitivity to noise and to painful stimuli. Further confirmation is that niacin deficiency as observed in pellagra, produces exactly these same symptoms along with more serious ones.

Are we safe in concluding that every individual who is irritable or difficult to get along with, is suffering from a specific lack of an amino acid, thiamin, or niacin? By no means. We cannot say for sure that deficient nutrition of any sort is necessarily involved. Yet the demonstrated facts lead us to wonder whether the very best nutrition of the entire nervous system would not help to eliminate from the lives of many people these unfortunate attitudes which border on disease. Certainly if a small infant is peevish and cries excessively we are led to suspect that something may be wrong with the food. Why does not the same principle apply to adults? To accept this possibility does not deny the existence of moral responsibility of adults and the ability of each individual to exert control over his own life. One of the responsibilities he has, incidentally, is to eat as wisely as he can.

Problems involving the nervous system include the loss of memory; this also may have a nutritional cause. Korsakoff's syndrome and Wernicke's disease, both of which involve loss of memory and mental confusion, are thought to be due to nutritional deficiencies of long standing, and some cases have responded well to nutritional therapy. Senile dementia which is also associated with loss of memory (particularly for recent events) probably has as its fundamental cause the failure of the partially clogged blood vessels to bring adequate nourishment to the brain cells.

Another problem that may have a nutritional basis is that of insomnia or sleeplessness. Deficiencies of minerals, calcium, and potassium, for example, tend to produce insomnia as do also deficiencies of vitamin B_1, vitamin B_6, niacin, and perhaps others. Sleeping is a normal function and the fact that it can be interfered with by nutritional inadequacies suggests the probability that it is often the result of inadequate nourishment of the nerve cells. That sleep has a physiological basis (one which involves cells and tissues) is amply demonstrated whenever one successfully uses sleeping pills. These, of course, induce sleep by drug action which is quite a different thing from inducing sleep by furnishing the nerve cells a needed nutrient with which they have been inadequately supplied.

An ailment that involves nerves and may have a nutritional basis is headache. Of course there are headaches and headaches; they probably have a multitude of origins and all types cannot be discussed in the same breath. Many medical reports tell of cases where headache has been relieved or abolished by attention to nutrition and I, personally, have known individuals who said that severe daily headaches were promptly eliminated when they began taking a nutritional supplement. The number of suggestions along this line are sufficiently large so that one who is subject to headaches may well wonder whether or not there is a nutritional cause that can be eliminated.

Severe mental depression and actual insanity can be brought about by nutritional deficiency. The most striking examples of this are to be found in the disease pellagra which has sometimes been described as exhibiting the "three D's"—dermatitis, diarrhea, and dementia. The psychological symptoms often involve vivid imaginings, persecutions, and, finally, complete withdrawal so that the victim pays no attention whatever to what doctors or nurses may say. Such cases have been almost miraculously cured within a period of 48 hours by the administration of the principal missing nutrient, niacinamide. As a result of such administration the individual may become completely coherent, may remember the past "craziness" and be extremely gratified that the array of crazy ideas now makes no sense. Even a wildly delirious victim of pellagra may sometimes within 36 hours become calm and rational after being given a good dose of the missing vitamin. This particular vitamin is one of those absolutely essential for brain metabolism.

While it would be rash indeed to conclude from these well-established facts that insanity is always caused by niacinamide lack—this is not true—it is quite reasonable to speculate that in many insanities inadequate nerve-cell nutrition may play an important role. That insanity has a physiological basis (involving cells and tissues) is becoming more and more apparent in recent years when the use of drugs has demonstrated that something close to insanity can be produced by some drugs, and in many cases insanity can be relieved by other drugs. Drug treatment, when it works, is better than no treatment at all, but nutritional treatment and prevention when it becomes available will be a vast improvement.

To emphasize that insanity has a physiological basis is, of course, not to deny the existence of psychological influences. Mental attitudes and emotions affect one's body chemistry, and one's training and experience, and the way one governs one's life all have a bearing on how one's physiology functions. In this area as well as others "ideas have consequences."

Other diseases involving nerve structures that might be approached from the nutritional angle are: epilepsy, multiple sclerosis, muscular dystrophy, and *paralysis agitans* (palsy).

Certainly none of these diseases is simple, and nutritional treatments that can be counted on to work are not available. Only certain individuals are susceptible to these diseases, and the diseases are almost certainly associated with peculiarities in the cellular metabolism of the susceptible individuals. Some of these afflictions have, in individual cases, been treated nutritionally with success and there is hope that progress will result from further investigation along the lines of cellular nutrition and the complications that arise from it.

Up to now we have not mentioned one of the most important killers of all—cancer. Can this problem by any chance have a nutritional basis?

It would take us too far afield to discuss cancer in any detail, so we will limit ourselves to a few pertinent statements. If cancer cells required for their nutrition an assortment of nutrients quite different from those required by normal cells, then it should be possible by judicious selection and use of nutrients to starve out the cancer cells and maintain the healthy ones. Unfortunately, cancer cells need for their nutrition *about the same nutrients* as other cells. As a result, if one wishes to starve cancer cells—this can be done— the normal cells are starved also and the results are worthless. Success in directly combating cancer cells depends upon finding some peculiarities in their metabolism which will make them vulnerable to nutritional lacks or to specific poisons which do not kill normal cells.

Evidence is accumulating rapidly which indicates that many cancers—probably all cancers—arise because of viruslike agents that invade normal cells. Well-nourished cells are, in general, relatively resistant to outside attack, and one of the strong hopes for *prevention* of cancer lies in the field of specialized nutrition. This, again, is by no means a simple matter but certainly the outlook in this direction is not hopeless.

In this chapter we have presented evidence that many diseases of many different types affecting many different cells and tissues, may have a nutritional basis. Indeed, whenever increased blood supply is induced in any part of the body by the use, for example, of hot packs, foot baths, or sitz baths, much of the benefit is no doubt derived from the better nutrition of the tissues which receive the improved blood supply.

Anyone who imagines that he or she, utilizing nutritional knowledge, knows how to treat all types of diseases is suffering from self-delusion. It is not that simple, and nutritional knowledge does not yet make this possible. The material we have presented is extremely suggestive, however, and there can be no intelligent doubt that nutrition holds out many possibilities for the successful treatment and prevention of a great variety of diseases. Nutritional science is on the threshold of tremendous new developments.

VI

How Common Is Deficient Nutrition?

History tells us that ever since Biblical times there have been periodic famines in various areas of the world where crop failures have made it impossible for people to get enough to eat. Population explosions in relatively lush years have resulted in overtaxing the food-producing economies of the affected regions in lean years. Available calories are limited, bodily reserves are exhausted, and emaciation results. This kind of deficient nutrition is relatively easy to recognize; its causes are obvious and it is rare in the U.S.A.

Other forms of deficient nutrition are those in which food calories are not necessarily limited, but the quality of the food is such as to promote overt disease. One of the outstanding examples of this type of deficient nutrition involves the too-exclusive use of polished rice and induces the disease beriberi. Millions of people have died from this disease which, unfortunately, has been far from eradicated. Of course, poverty and limited access to diversified foods have been factors in the production of this disease, but the basic lack is not calories; rather the victims get biochemically about one-fourth as much thiamin (vitamin B_1) as they need. If people get *no* thiamin at all they die before they have time to contract the disabling disease.

Other prominent diseases that are recognized to be due to specific nutritional lacks are pellagra (niacinamide lack, primarily), scurvy (vitamin C lack), rickets (often a lack of vitamin D), and kwashiorkor (inadequate protein). Actual cases of these diseases are often more complicated than might appear on the surface, because different nutritional lacks often come together, and an individual might quite conceivably be affected simultaneously with mild deficiencies of several kinds as well as diseases with infectious origins.

Since this little book is primarily for American consumption and these overt diseases do not occur frequently in our country, we are concerned in this chapter with the kind of deficient nutrition which may impair health, vigor, and well-being without generating any one of these clinically well-recognized deficiency diseases.

First let us consider the problem of such deficiencies in our animals. Since we are likely to feed our animals about as effectively as we do ourselves (often more so), we can get a partial answer from this source.

When I was in my early teens I embarked upon a venture involving nutrition that looked most promising, but did not live up to its promise. I could buy baby chicks at the then going price of five cents each and after feeding them for a few weeks I could sell them as broilers for about forty cents apiece. What nicer way could there be for turning $5.00 into $40.00 or even $10.00 into $80.00? So I built some pens at small expense and went into the business in a modest way, commensurate with my available capital.

Unfortunately, at that time I had no knowledge about what I am writing now. I entertained the same vague notions about nutrition that so many of my countrymen still appear to hold. I knew that the chicks had to eat, I had some idea of how much they would eat, but I had little idea as to the quality; consequently I simply fed them grain in abundance. Failure in my venture was forthcoming; so many chicks died that my anticipated profits vanished into thin air. The principal cause of death was, as I now know, malnutrition, in which quality was lacking even though quantity was not.

Much is now known about the nutrition of baby chicks which no one knew at that time. If chicks do not, *from the start*, get *plenty* of every mineral, amino acid, and vitamin they need, their nervous appetite mechanism is starved sufficiently so it ceases to function. They stop eating and die. For many years chicks were not used as experimental animals in nutrition investigations for this very reason. Experimental diets of known composition could not be concocted that would keep their appetites in working order. It was only after the discovery of a substantial number of vitamins, that baby chicks could be raised successfully on diets of known composition.

About ten years after the chicken project, I had occasion to do a nutritional experiment with rats for the company for which I worked as a research biochemist. I purchased from an animal dealer in Chicago about thirty young weanling white rats and provided individual cages for them. With seeming innocence I asked the animal dealer what to feed the young rats. He sold me a large bag of coarse meal which he said emphatically was *just the thing*. It contained ground-up seeds of various kinds including a few sunflower seeds. Before starting the rats on the experiment, I kept them under observation for a week and fed them exactly as directed by the experienced animal dealer. I kept an exact record of their individual weights because in a rat at this stage of development, growth as determined by weight gain, is a crucial criterion of well-being. After the first week I knew just how much each rat had grown, and I placed all of them on experimental diets of my own concoction. In spite of the fact that my concocted diets were purposely deficient in some respects, the rats—somewhat to my surprise—grew almost exactly twice as fast the second week as they had the previous week on the animal dealer's food. This was, of course, a short-term experiment; my diets would not have shown superiority over a long period.

The conclusion was inevitable: the animal dealer's diet was a deficient one; for a short period at least they would have done better on my diet; his animals were regularly suffering from mild malnutrition based on poor quality. Not only this, but the state of nutritional science at the time this experiment was done was such that no animal dealer anywhere knew how to feed young animals qualitatively well, according to present-day standards. From my present knowledge about the diets used, it is clear that what the rats lacked on the animal dealer's food was an adequate assortment of amino acids. My experimental diets, though deficient in some other ways that would have shown up in longer term experiments, were well supplied with high-quality protein which yielded the animals an excellent assortment of beads (amino acids) from which to build their proteins.

The deficient nutrition in the case of the animal dealer's rats was not as severe as that experienced by my baby chicks ten years before, because the rats did live and would eventually be able to propagate. The nutritional needs of these weanling rats (which were about 8 weeks old counting from the time of conception) were far less exacting than those of baby chicks which are embryologically only 3 weeks old when they hatch. Newborn rats probably have needs about as exacting as that of baby chicks, but, of course, for 3 weeks or more they live on their mother's milk, and during this time their reserves are built up and their needs become less exacting.

Weight gain in young animals has been traditionally the most often used criterion for well-being. If a young animal grows, this is a sign that it is getting what it needs in its food. This criterion is a highly convenient one to apply and has been used many thousands of times in nutritional investigations. It is not, however, without its drawbacks and question marks. How rapidly, for example, should a rat (the most commonly used experimental animal) grow during the post-weanling stage? In the early history of nutritional studies, it was concluded that if such a rat grew at the rate of about a gram a day (an ounce a month) it was nourished satisfactorily. This is about what the animal dealer expected though he did not put his expectations in these terms.

A few years later, as nutritional knowledge increased, there was a gradual increase in the expected growth rate of rats. Not many years later, a gain of two grams a day was considered very satisfactory. All of this sounds rather ridiculous now, because we know that well-nourished growing rats—given plenty of all the amino acids, minerals, and vitamins now known to be needed—will gain weight at the rate of 5 or 6 grams a day or even more!

Another question raises its head here. Is it best for rats (or children) that they grow very rapidly? For example, do rats live longer if they are given diets that make them grow rapidly? The answer to this question is not clear cut, but it seems unlikely that longevity can be assured by continuously furnishing abundant amounts of a good growth-promoting ration. There are complications which we will discuss shortly.

This brings us to another criterion that can be used to test the value of a diet, namely, ability to reproduce. For this type of experiment it is obviously necessary to carry the animals along for generations; this extends the length of experiments and increases the cost due to the expense of feeding and caring for the animals. Dr. Henry Clapp Sherman and his coworkers at Columbia University were among the first to carry out such experiments about 35 years ago. They found, for example, that a mixture of ⅙ whole-milk powder and ⅚ ground whole wheat with added salt and water constituted a diet on which rats could reproduce for many generations. On this diet, weanling rats gained on the average about 1.5 grams a day. The total number of young reared by female rats on this diet averaged less than six during their reproductive lifetime, whereas when the proportion of whole-milk powder was increased to ¼ and the ground whole wheat was decreased to ¾, the individual female rats reared, on an average, 18 young. Even this is a puny record; we have in our laboratory well-fed female rats which can readily rear in a lifetime well over 100 young.

Still another criterion of well-being that can be used to evaluate a diet is length of life. This involves long-drawn-out experiments and obviously it is impractical with ordinary animal quarters and without inordinate expense to carry out tests on all kinds of diets, using longevity as a criterion. Sherman and co-workers found that their rats on the ⅙ milk-⅚ wheat diet lived on an average of 587 days whereas on the ¼ milk-¾ wheat mixture they lived 652 days. This was an 11 per cent increase in life span and on the human scale would mean 7 or 8 years.

In our laboratories we have recently carried out an experiment involving longevity as the criterion, using mice as the experimental animal. We fed all the mice a commercial animal chow compounded with modern knowledge and containing a supposed abundance of everything that mice need. In other words, the *quality* of the diet was high—probably it was higher in quality than most pets get and certainly higher in quality than most humans consume. That it was a superior diet is indicated by the fact that the mice receiving it, and nothing else, lived an average of 549.8 days, nearly as long as the rats on Sherman's ⅙ milk-⅚ wheat diet—this in spite of the fact that mice usually live only about three-fourths as long as rats. To a parallel group of mice we added in their drinking water—this was the only difference—enough pantothenate so that the animals received about 0.3 mg. of pantothenate extra per day beyond that in the animal chow. The mice receiving the additional pantothenate lived an average of 653.1 days—one day longer than the *rats* on Sherman's improved diet. This was an average increase of over 18 per cent and on the human scale would have meant an increased life span of about 13 years.

Deficient nutrition is exemplified in these various experiments. My baby chicks died of severe malnutrition—their appetite mechanisms failed before they had time to exhibit disease. The animal dealer's rats suffered from inadequate amounts of the various amino acids (and probably from other deficiencies also). Sherman's rats on the ⅙ milk-⅚ wheat diet suffered from deficient nutrition because, when the diet was improved by making it ¼ milk and ¾ wheat, the condition of the animals, as judged by several criteria, was markedly improved. Even the ¼ milk-¾ wheat diet was substantially deficient and could be improved further by additional vitamins and minerals. Rats on this diet had a low reproductive record and gained less than 3 grams per day which is well below optimal. Even the modern commercial animal chow fed to our mice was a deficient one, because the animals lived nearly 20 per cent longer when *additional* pantothenate was given.

An interesting and complicating wrinkle exists with respect to all longevity experiments; this is the question of the *quantity* of food consumed. Dr. Clive McCay at Cornell University made the striking discovery many years ago that rats with limited food intake live much longer than if they always have access to all they want. Rats can be kept in a "juvenile" state for two years by underfeeding them; then if they are fed at a higher level they will grow and become adult and, finally, senescent. The period of senescence can be greatly delayed, however, by underfeeding. To promote long life in rats one may feed them very high quality food but give them continuously less than they will eat. It seems probable that restricted intake during early youth would be less advantageous than restriction later in life. A continuous abundance of high-quality food obtained without effort is not conducive to longevity in rats.

The implications of these findings for humans are not crystal clear. Rats continue to grow over a large part of their life span, and in this way differ from human beings who may often live, after they cease to grow, three or four times as long as their "growth period." People often respond to the results of Dr. McCay by asking the question, "Who wants to live a long and hungry life?" His findings are extremely suggestive, however, that adult human beings are harmed more by over-eating than by undereating. Religious or other fasts of short duration may be physiologically beneficial. Dr. George Crile, a famed surgeon, made a statement years ago to the effect that Americans, by overeating, dig their own graves with their teeth.

Using the criteria of (1) growth of young animals, (2) ability to reproduce, and (3) longevity, it becomes clear from these and other experiments that, among animals in general, deficient nutrition must be very common indeed.

There are, however, other criteria of well-being besides those already mentioned. One of these which we have been investigating is vigor or "peppiness." Our means of testing animals for this involves giving them access to an exercise wheel to play in that records all revolutions of the wheel—forward or backward. In a recent experiment which must be repeated on a larger scale, we obtained some surprisingly interesting results.

Animals (rats) were given diets with the following characteristics:

A—adequate
B—adequate except vitamin B₁ missing
C—adequate except pyridoxin missing
D—adequate except pantothenate missing

Using growth as a criterion of well-being the animals on diets B and C showed definite malnourishment within each of the first two weeks, in that growth was diminished. On diet D, however, the pantothenate deficiency did not make itself known by an immediate decrease in growth rate. Using peppiness as a criterion, the situation was reversed. The tendency of the rats to play on the exercise wheels was about the same on diets A, B, and C. The deficiencies of vitamin B_1 or of pyridoxin did not immediately diminish the desire of the rats to exercise. On diet D, however, where pantothenate deficiency existed, there was in the two-week period a significant decrease in the desire to exercise. Subject to further verification, it appears that pantothenate deficiency may tend to make animals sluggish and pepless. If this is so, the early use of the exercise wheel in nutritional studies might have made pantothenate one of the first vitamins to be discovered.

It is not to be presumed that the exercise wheel is an infallible test for peppiness. It may be there are more contemplative ways in which rats (or humans) can be peppy that would not show up in this test. It is, however, one way by which we can get a hint as to an animal's internal vigor.

Another criterion of well-being in rats is stamina. How much stamina a rat has at a particular time can be ascertained, for example, by spinning the rat in an exercise wheel and noting when he becomes exhausted and unable to run longer. Another means of determining stamina is to force the animal to swim until exhausted (and then rescue it before it drowns) and note the swimming time. It is by this means that it has been found recently that the amino acid, aspartic acid, is possibly of greater nutritional importance than has been previously suspected. Administering salts of aspartic acid to rats is reported to double the length of time they can swim before exhaustion! Corroboration of this increase in stamina has been reported in the case of human beings (athletes) also. These results are more impressive because there appear to be sound biochemical reasons why aspartates might have this effect. However, further confirmation is necessary.

There are a number of other criteria of well-being that might be used for testing the adequacy of diets if they were not so time consuming and expensive. Rats on deficient diets do not develop well mentally, as judged, for example, by maze-running ability. It is conceivable that this might be used as a criterion of excellent nutrition and that deficiencies might be discovered by this means that would not be readily apparent otherwise. Ability to remember (how to run in a maze, for example) could be used in the same way. In human beings there is no question that in some cases (Korsakoff's syndrome, for example), failure of memory is associated with nutritional deficiency. Visual abilities might also be used in the same way. It is well known that vision is affected adversely by deficient nutrition. The maintenance of normal electroencephalographs (brain waves) might also be used. Some of my colleagues have recently found that, in chicks, each of several types of deficiencies produces different and characteristic abnormalities in brain-wave patterns.

Still another kind of criterion can be used. It has been observed in many laboratories, including ours, that rats on high-quality diets voluntarily consume far less alcohol (also less sugar) than those on deficient diets. In individual rats it has been possible to shift their alcohol consumption up and down at will by deliberately making them deficient in specific vitamins, and then supplying the missing nutrients. This involves the loss or gain of body wisdom, which may exhibit itself in other ways. The failure to develop obesity (in experimental animals) might be used as a criterion of well-being and highly developed body wisdom. Presumably the best diet for an animal would be one which would be least conducive to the production of obesity.

When we consider the many criteria for well-being that might be used to evaluate diets (many of which have not been developed), it becomes clearly evident that the very best nutrition for animals, whether laboratory rats, household pets or livestock, is far from established and that deficient nutrition of a type that causes no overt deficiency disease must be very common.

Next let us turn to human beings. To what extent prenatal nutritional deficiencies may play a role in abnormalities and ill health may be judged from the contents of the previous chapter. Let us ask this question about babies: Are they, in the U.S.A., always or usually nourished at a level of excellence such as not to retard development or contribute to ill health in later years? I think it can be said without equivocation that babies are better cared for nutritionally than any other segment of the population—at least more attention is paid to their nutrition. Babies are never offered a breakfast of sweet rolls and coffee or pancakes and syrup, nor do they have the opportunity to eat a lunch consisting of a hamburger accompanied by a beverage of well-sweetened carbonated water.

Those young infants who get milk from a well-nourished mother, undoubtedly are nourished very well indeed. This does not mean that they should not be encouraged to supplement this diet with fruits, vegetables, meats, etc., at an early age. The use of modified cow's milk as a substitute for mother's milk during early infancy is a practical one which often seems to yield good results. It is, however, a substitute and as such is inferior. How inferior modified cow's milk is for very young babies is not fully known, though relatively recent statistics from England and Sweden indicate that there is a substantially lower death rate and sickness rate in babies that are breast fed. It is reasonable that the proportions of minerals, amino acids, and vitamins most suitable for calves would not have the highest suitability for babies.

In recent years Dr. Paul György of Philadelphia has shown that human milk contains a vitamin-like nutrient which is almost absent from cow's milk. The exact significance of this substance is not clear. Its function may be to modify the bacterial contents of the baby's intestinal tract; it is known to be necessary for the nutrition of certain harmless bacteria. It is also possible that it is used directly by the tissues of the growing infant.

That deficient nutrition of the type which does not lead to clinically defined deficiency diseases has been common among children has been demonstrated many times by the simple expedient of adding more milk to the diet of school children. Such children improve in health, performance, and spirits and in every other way. The results have been striking enough so that the use of extra milk in school-lunch programs has been widely adopted and generally approved. The trial use of vitamin and other supplements has also shown that children often benefit from such additions to their diet. That even rickets (often in mild form) is not uncommon in children who are supposedly well fed is shown by the fact that Dr. Edwards Park found among 230 post-mortems on children (about 1940) that almost half (107) showed histological signs of the disease. No informed person can doubt that the nutrition of almost any group of school children could be improved today by the inclusion of more wholesome food including milk and dairy products.

That deficient nutrition is to be found commonly among adults (even among those who regard themselves well nourished) can hardly be doubted in light of all the facts we have set forth with respect to animal nutrition and the types of ills that can be caused by faulty nutrition (Chapter V). Nearly twenty years ago a committee of the National Research Council reported on this subject and concluded that inadequate diets and deficiency states are widespread through the nation. The situation has not changed materially during the intervening years. The statement has even more justification (on the basis of better insights) than it had when it was made.

We have already referred to the experiment in a tuberculosis hospital where patients were already said to be "exceedingly well nourished," but were nevertheless markedly benefited by nutritional supplements. Certainly if the patients who did not receive the supplements got well more slowly as a result and failed to keep their appetites, to make satisfactory weight gains, and were unable to look after their minor needs, they were suffering from deficient nutrition.

One segment of the population which is perhaps peculiarly susceptible to deficient nutrition includes those in the elderly or past-middle-age bracket. The rationale behind this probability is that during the period of aging, particular cells, tissues, and organs begin to show wear and tear which, theoretically at least, can be delayed by furnishing these structures with highest-quality nutrition. In a book published in England in 1961, *Recent Advances in Nutrition* by J. F. Brock, the opinion is stressed by competent authorities that a large proportion of old people are poorly nourished and that the vitamin needs of older people are substantially higher than those of other adults.

There is a real question as to whether in the human experiments that have been performed (in the tuberculosis hospital referred to above and elsewhere), the supplements used have been chosen with expert care. This problem will be discussed in a later chapter of this book. This uncertainty does not detract from the fact that many experiments and observations point to deficient nutrition as at least a contributing cause of human difficulties. Almost any segment of the human population can have its nutrition improved, especially if we were to use as criteria of well-being not only growth (of children), but also reproduction, longevity, peppiness, stamina, mental vigor, and body wisdom. Deficient nutrition, at least of a mild sort, must be extremely common.

This concept of deficient nutrition—which may be of all degrees from mild to severe—is entirely in keeping with what we have had to say about cellular nutrition. Cells and tissues can be nourished at various levels of efficiency; whole animals can be nourished with food of all degrees of quality. Failure in nutrition may adversely affect any or every function of our bodies.

Potentially, at least, there is quite a different type of factor in modern life which is capable of contributing to deficient nutrition. This is the extensive use of pesticides in the never-ending war between human beings and insects and other pests. Because of the unity of nature, already discussed, the poisons we use in fighting insects are capable of backfiring on us. Effective poisons usually affect the enzymes in the organism that is poisoned. An ideal insect poison would be one that knocks out the insect enzymes and leaves our own enzymes unaffected. Such an ideal is difficult or impossible to reach; no insect poison can with safety be administered in substantial doses to human beings.

The quantitative aspects are all important in this connection. One cannot use arsenic sprays for the control of codling moth on apple trees, and at the same time make it possible for people to eat apples without getting a few atoms (p. 25) of arsenic in their systems. The important thing is to hold the spray residues to such a level that people will not get sufficient arsenic to do any damage. Arsenic is in all our bodies in small amounts and has been since before arsenic sprays were invented. The possibility is not ruled out that arsenic may be a trace element essential for our well-being. It is important for our health, however, that we not get too much.

The situation with respect to the elements copper and cobalt is somewhat similar. These are violent poisons if used in too large amounts, but traces are absolutely essential to life. The quantitative aspects of the problem are paramount.

Sometimes we hear "nature enthusiasts" object to the use of DDT for insect control on the basis that it is a poison and the traces we get are bound to poison us, cause cancer, and do all sorts of damage. Here the quantitative aspects of the problem stand out. The crucial question is: Are we likely to get *enough* DDT to hurt us (assuming we do not eat DDT-killed flies) under the prevailing conditions of use? Conservation of all forms of bird life simultaneous with the extensive use of insect poisons presents a special problem because insects are an important food for birds.

The extensive corps of experts who have charge of the control of the use of pesticides are acquainted with all these problems. While they may sometimes make mistakes, they make a sincere effort to guard health, and I would rather trust the control to their hands than I would to the inexpert and uninformed individuals who often become very vocal on the subject.

The old saying "You can't have your cake and eat it too," applies to this situation. It would be nice if we could always be free from insects when we want to without using insect poisons, but wormless apples and insect sprays go together; if you avoid all insect sprays you can eat wormy apples (provided you can get to them before they rot). Many people like all the advantages of living under sanitary conditions, at the same time they hark back to the good old days and the practices that made sanitation impossible. A fact which is bound to affect human lives all over the world is the existence of tremendously increasing numbers of human beings. Primitive living under idyllic conditions is incompatible with world population as it is and will be in the decades to come. If we are insistent on back-to-nature living, we are in effect advocating an elimination of a large proportion of the human race. A better perspective involves recognizing human beings, including their reproduction and their chemical and other ingenuity, as a part of nature. Instead of back to nature, a better slogan might be "forward with nature."

The use of pesticides is and must be controlled. If there is failure here, the offending agents may modify the working of our enzymes, which in turn may modify our nutritional needs and render satisfactory nutrition more difficult. It is important that the control of the use of pesticides be in the hands of qualified experts and that they not be harassed by those whose background knowledge is too limited to allow them to make wise judgments.

VII

Nutrition Education
in the National Interest

It is vitally important from the standpoint of both public and private health that education and research in nutrition be promoted at an accelerated pace. Research *must* accompany education. It would be unthinkable that we should be content to teach merely what we now know when such attractive and rewarding frontiers lie immediately ahead to be explored.

The two outstanding frontiers include: first, cellular nutrition with all its implications and applications; and second, the relation of genetics to nutrition and to the needs of individuals.

In this small volume we have already called attention to the important fact that nutrition is not only for the body as a whole but for its multitude of parts—the cells and tissues that make it up. Also the fact that the nutrition of particular cells is not only derived from the chemicals in the food that we eat but also from chemicals produced by other body cells and brought to the recipient cells by the circulating blood. Certain cells in our bodies may be, to a degree, parasitic on other cells. Yet our knowledge about this whole scheme is vague and unsatisfactory. There is much fundamental information about this basic phase of nutrition that is now beyond our ken.

The relationship between genetics and nutrition is no less

alluring and potentially productive. Over twenty years ago, pioneering investigation showed a close relationship between genes, the carriers of inheritance, and the enzymes which we have earlier discussed. It was only recently that these outstanding findings were recognized by the awarding of Nobel prizes to the pioneer investigators (Beadle and Tatum). Even today, the full implications of this work are not appreciated by many. If genes are the "fathers" of enzymes as this work showed, then since each individual has a distinctive assortment of genes, it follows that the enzyme patterns of each person is distinctive. This means, in turn, that in the quantitative sense each person has a distinctive pattern of nutritional needs.

Direct experiment has already indicated with respect to amino acids that some individual persons require two, four, or six times as much of a particular amino acid as others do for maintenance of health. This is a reflection of differences (of genetic origin) in the effectiveness of our various enzymes. There are also many similar indications with respect to other nutrients. This is too large a subject to be discussed in detail here. Enough has been said to indicate how important it is to know more about these differences in need and to what extent the old saying is true: "What is one man's meat is another's poison."

To be content to teach merely what we have already learned about nutrition would be as ridiculous as invoking a moratorium on new discoveries in the area of atomic energy while teaching oncoming generations only the accumulative knowledge of past decades. In stressing the importance of education (and inevitable research) in nutrition, we may well pause to ask, "Who needs to be educated?" The answer is simple: everybody.

I am not one of those intellectual snobs who underrates people in general, and their ability to grasp important facts. I do not know or care about the abilities of some hypothetical average person who does not exist. I do know that there are millions of intelligent people in our country who would profit by a better understanding of nutrition. Actually, support for education and research comes from the public. If the public is not aware of the possibilities, support will not be forthcoming. So it is essential that the public, including the oncoming generation of boys and girls, be educated as to nutrition and its present and future possibilities.

A second question may be asked, "Who are the experts who will ultimately furnish the insight that will make ongoing nutrition education possible?" The answer is relatively simple: *trained biochemists* who direct their attention to nutritional problems. Not only are all nutritional items *chemical* items, but the significant transformations that take place in our bodies involving these nutritional substances are *chemical* in nature. It is therefore obvious that an expert in the field of nutrition—regardless of what else he may know—must be at home in dealing with the complex chemical interrelationships between amino acids, minerals, vitamins, proteins, fats, carbohydrates, enzymes, hormones, nucleic acids, etc. Mere interest in nutrition—however great—cannot make one an expert unless he or she has sound chemical and biochemical knowledge and understanding.

A medical education has as its primary purpose the training of physicians. This generalized training does not in this day of greatly specialized knowledge, produce experts in nutrition. While medical students always take a substantial course in biochemistry early in their medical training, they also have on their minds many other subjects—anatomy, neurology, pathology, immunology, etc.—and do not specialize in biochemistry or in nutrition. During their medical training physicians-to-be gain a tremendous store of information and insight about human bodies and their functioning. They are thus in a peculiar position to appreciate the potentialities of nutrition, but without additional specialized training in nutritional biochemistry, they do not qualify as nutritional experts.

One reason why more education is needed by the public is so they will not be so gullible in the acceptance of faddist ideas. I think of five authors who have either local or even national reputations as "authorities" in the field of nutrition —some of their names have come to be almost household words; yet a recent perusal of *American Men of Science,* a series of volumes listing every reputable scientist in this country, revealed—not to my great surprise—that not one of these five "eminent nutrition authorities" is listed. Not only are they unqualified in biochemistry or nutrition, they are not even scientists in some related field.

I am certainly in favor of freedom in the publication of books. Even books on nutrition should not be censored. However, the public needs to be educated to the point where it will ask a supposed expert to show his credentials, before it accepts what he writes as authoritative or his opinions as worth serious consideration. Certainly I would not go so far as to say that nothing a relatively uninformed person can say about nutrition is true. Neither would I say that experts are absolutely infallible or that the mere possession of some kind of doctor's degree entitles one to speak authoritatively. Unfortunately a few members of the medical profession have in the past—and even in the present—taken advantage of people's gullibility and have presented prime foolishness in the guise of authoritative discussions. Too often books of this character have become best sellers.

Before this gullibility can be eliminated, the public needs to know that there have been tremendous developments in biochemistry during the past twenty years. It is common public knowledge that there has been an astounding revolution in the thinking of physicists and chemists with respect to atomic energy, and that an "expert" in this field of fifteen years ago could not talk intelligibly to an expert of today. It is not so well known that biochemistry has undergone a metamorphosis; a biochemical expert of today talks a different language from the expert of a decade or two ago. Biochemistry has also expanded so that there are experts in restricted areas who are inexpert so far as nutrition is concerned. Specialized knowledge is very much in vogue.

The growth of biochemistry has been phenomenal. In 1938, for the first time it appeared in tabulations as a separate branch of science. Since that time it has risen to take and maintain a position among the top four or five branches of science in which doctorate degrees are granted. Furthermore, it has permeated to a high degree many other branches of science: bacteriology, botany, zoology, genetics, etc. Times have changed so that what may have been true twenty years ago when biochemistry was a toddling infant no longer holds. Certainly it now encompasses a tremendous and highly complicated body of information and insight—far beyond what the medical student can be expected to assimilate.

The future relationships between medicine, biochemistry and nutrition are uncertain. It is no discredit to a proctologist that he is not an expert in otolaryngology; it is no discredit to a brain surgeon that he is not an expert allergist. It is no discredit whatsoever to the medical profession as a whole in the 1960's that they are not experts in biochemistry or in nutrition.

The opinion is frequently expressed that students do not get enough biochemical and nutritional education in medical schools. Some think that nutrition should be developed into a medical specialty like other specialties: urology, obstetrics, anesthesiology, etc. What will come in the future is unknown. The American Medical Association has a committee studying the subject. The way ahead is not perfectly clear; medical curricula are already crowded and there is a limit to what one may ask a prospective physician to learn.

One of the common-sense points of view that has resulted

from improved knowledge of biochemistry and nutrition, is the sharp distinction which should be made between the two types of remedial agents indicated below.

TYPE I	TYPE II
Remedial chemical agents foreign to our bodies and to natural food, but found (often by trial and error) to be more or less valuable in the treatment of disease.	Remedial chemical agents present in our bodies and in natural food. Potentially valuable because they enter constructively into metabolic machinery.

Aspirin, penicillin, and other antibiotics are outstanding examples of valuable remedial agents belonging in Type I. Type II remedial agents include not only the hormones (which are normally produced within our bodies) but such nutritional substances as lysine, glutamine, vitamin A, and the many others listed on pages 21–23.

Type I agents should be and have been used (with a few exceptions including aspirin which is judged safe) only on a doctor's prescription. Hormones, which normally are not food products, are and should be used only under a qualified doctor's supervision. The nutritional remedial agents of Type II, on the other hand, should not, and have not, required a physician's prescription. Exceptions may exist in rare cases where there may be danger that people will make too free use of the natural chemicals which may be available to druggists. These constructive remedial agents are food substances and while physicians often advise their patients what to eat, prescriptions for food are inappropriate and have never been used.

Because the development of biochemistry has been recent, there has been a lag in identifying biochemists as the experts who are to be trusted in nutritional matters. The Food and Drug Administration requires that on certain labels it must be stated with respect to various items contained in the package: NEED IN HUMAN NUTRITION NOT ESTABLISHED. Among the items so designated, is zinc. The question arises, "Who needs to be satisfied on this point before it can be said to be *established?*" Obviously, the experts. Clearly the man in the street is not one of those who should be consulted. Neither should those self-styled experts who have no scientific standing. A lawyer would not know the answer. The real experts are the biochemists who know most about the chemistry of living things and are perfectly at home with such problems.

Zinc, to discuss this particular example, is an indispensable constituent of an enzyme "carbonic anhydrase." This enzyme is in our bodies and needs to be there to hasten the decomposition of carbonic acid. The enzyme has to be made in our bodies, it cannot be made without zinc and the only way we can get the zinc is through nutrition. Therefore the need for zinc in human nutrition *has been established.* Perhaps it has not been established in the eyes of untutored individuals; if it is established in the eyes of the experts this should be enough. No competent biochemist can be found who has any doubt about the need for zinc in human nutrition.

One way to establish the need for zinc in human nutrition would be to feed human individuals a diet lacking zinc until illness overtook them, and then administer zinc as an effective cure of the illness. But this direct method is unnecessarily inhumane as well as very expensive. This direct demonstration is quite unnecessary to convince an expert, though it might be required to convince one who knows little about biochemistry. The need for phosphate in human nutrition (which *everyone* accepts) has never been demonstrated by feeding human beings everything but phosphate until they become ill, and then curing them with phosphate. This could be done, but it is not necessary in view of all that biochemists know about phosphate biochemistry.

Another item that falls in the same general category with zinc is the vitamin pantothenic acid (there are several others). Though there have been human experiments indicating the need for pantothenic acid, no one has applied the simple direct method of feeding a pantothenic-acid-free diet to human beings until they become ill, and then curing them by pantothenate administration. Because of the absence of this simple direct demonstration, the Food and Drug Administration rules that bottles containing this vitamin must bear a label indicating: NEED IN HUMAN NUTRITION NOT ESTABLISHED.

Experts who are acquainted with the functioning of coenzyme A (which contains this vitamin) in the whole biological kingdom and in all oxygen-using organisms in particular, do not need such a demonstration. A competent biochemist cannot be found who would express doubt as to need in human nutrition for this vitamin. So far as the experts are concerned, the need for pantothenate in human nutrition *has been established*. The opinion of the experts is all that matters.

I would not want to have any part in an experiment involving feeding human beings a pantothenate-free diet. It might turn out like the experiment with dogs in which they appeared reasonably well until a day or two before they suddenly died.

One factor in this situation, which is a relatively recent development, involves the appreciation of the unity of nature discussed in Chapter IV. In the early days of nutritional science it was *hoped* that experiments with animals would lead to knowledge about human nutrition. Now, in the light of tremendous advance in knowledge of how organisms are related to each other biochemically, we *know* that animal experiments, reasonably interpreted, are valid. If we find a particular vitamin to be needed by rats, mice, foxes, monkeys, hogs, dogs, cattle, horses, chickens, ducks, and turkeys (as is true of pantothenic acid), one can wager heavily without any further information, that it is needed by human beings as well. Experts have a growing appreciation of the unity of nature, of the validity of animal experiments, and their ability to translate them into human terms.

One of the normal sources whereby practicing physicians

keep abreast of new developments in all areas, are the pharmaceutical and drug houses which continually have new products to sell. It is practically impossible for a practicing physician to spend hours each day reading medical journals and he welcomes the opportunity to learn quickly about new developments from reputable firms he has learned to trust.

The Food and Drug Administration is in the process of developing a very hard-boiled attitude toward such firms—a policy which, despite its good intentions, is questioned from the standpoint of public interest. Such firms are prohibited from sending literature or digests of medical findings to doctors regarding any of their "unapproved" products, even though these reports tell the negative as well as the positive side of the story. This cuts off an important source of continued education for practicing physicians who need to be informed about new things and are intelligent enough to pass judgment for themselves. They do not need to be "protected" by the Food and Drug Administration in this manner.

In order for a new drug to be approved for sale it must pass strict barriers. This in itself is good but, unfortunately, the barriers are not always constructed with due appreciation of all the facts. For example, before a hitherto unused remedial agent (*even of Type II*) can be brought to the attention of physicians in an effective way, there must be obtained results of a statistically valid nature, demonstrating its value. This regulation, which at first glance, may seem fair, flies in the face of newer knowledge of the relation between genes and enzymes and the undeniable and potent possibility that some remedial agents are of value but not of universal value because of genetic differences between individuals.

If a remedial agent, especially of Type II, is valuable for 10 or 20 per cent of cases, physicians are entitled to know this and to act accordingly; possibly a patient they desperately want to help will be among the 10–20 per cent. Such a remedial agent as this may be extremely valuable in some cases and yet not yield statistical evidence of its worth.

Carefully regulated sale of agents of doubtful remedial value has real justification, but a sharp distinction should be made particularly between remedial agents of Type I and the nutritional substances of Type II. Agents which are foreign to the body should have to go through a careful scrutiny before their sale is allowed. An agent like lysine, on the other hand, is one that we must take into our bodies every day, and no possible harm can come from a moderate increase in the amount we consume. There is good evidence, which experts regard as conclusive, that bread protein would be markedly improved if an appropriate amount of lysine were added to it. Yet the Food and Drug Administration denies the right of manufacturers to put the natural chemical lysine into bread and still call it simply bread or enriched bread. Type I agents and the nutritional chemicals of Type II have an entirely different status in the eyes of experts. This needs to be recognized.

It should be remembered that the manufacture and sale of drugs, amino acids, vitamins, and the like, are legitimate businesses that serve human needs. Such businesses should receive from those who are interested in public health, more encouragement than is given to the tobacco business, the liquor business, the candy business, and the soft-drink business. These other businesses that make a negative or doubtful contribution to public health are permitted to advertise and sell their products freely. Candy, soft-drink, and liquor manufacturers are not compelled, for example, to indicate on labels the calorie content of their products—a bit of information highly pertinent to the problem of how much (or how little) should be consumed.

Food manufacturers need, I believe, to take on added responsibility for the nutritional value of the products they sell. They should have experts in the forefront of nutritional science who can help them produce products that are not only tasty and salable but nutritiously beneficial. To one who is versed in nutrition the T.V. chatter about the "good things" that are offered as food for children and adults, for breakfast and for other meals, is far from convincing. There is far too much attention to *sweet* things that are relatively easy to sell but are questionable nutritionally. There is often also, a lack of appreciation of sound nutritional ideas which have been generated in the last ten years. Here then, among food manufacturers, further education is also needed.

Education regarding nutritional science is an important health measure. It must stem from trained biochemists and must circulate freely not only among the general public but also to pharmacists, physicians, public-health authorities, food manufacturers and others who hold our good health in their hands.

VIII

Good Nutritional Advice

Nutrition would be simpler than it is if the old adage were strictly true: "The proof of the pudding is in the eating." The proof is not only in the eating but also in the subsequent metabolic effects. Because of this, expert advice about nutrition is in order. The "eating" can take care of itself.

This is a free country and advice is something that can be taken or left. The suggestions given in this chapter are offered in this spirit. Fundamentally, we have the right to choose for ourselves. If, for example, someone prefers to eat heartily, grow fat, and "enjoy life as long as it lasts," then this is his right and certainly no one is in a position to deny it.

Advice is easy to give, but my aim is higher than this. I want to give *good* advice. If I become too specific about *exactly* what, when, and how one should eat or should not eat, I am liable to fall into the error of giving "reversible" advice—good for some, bad for others. People's stomachs vary in size over about a six-fold range and each person's whole digestive, assimilative, and metabolic apparatus is sufficiently different so that such advice as, "Eat more roughage" or "Eat less frequently" or "Eat a heavy breakfast" may be of the reversible kind. There are people who should eat *less* roughage, there are those who should eat *more* frequently, and those whose systems call, under their living conditions, for a light breakfast. Recommendation of specific food articles (such as sauerkraut or asparagus) may also be reversible. There are those who should leave sauerkraut or asparagus alone. A faddist usually thinks everyone should eat just as he eats. I am not a faddist.

Although each of us is a distinctive individual with distinctive needs, there is some advice which is applicable to all. For people in general, I will list these pieces of advice under five main headings.

I. *Don't be a hypochondriac or a worry wart.* Maybe if you are reasonably well and youthful enough for your age you ought to eat about as you do already and thank God for your good health. Worry and concern (about anything, including your health) can help unhinge what good health you have and can make a good nutritional situation deteriorate into a bad one. Worry is able to alter the working of our body chemistry so that the demands for specific nutrients may become augmented. Experimental animals put under stress need, for example, an increased supply of pantothenate to keep their bodily machinery working properly.

There is probably no such thing as nutrition which is perfect in every respect, and undue striving for absolute perfection may have an unfortunate effect. Some people's idea of an ideal community would be one in which there are plenty of doctors and hospitals to which one can run for every ache and pain, at all times—day and night. My idea of an ideal community would be one in which good doctors and hospitals are available but seldom needed—only for real emergencies. Physicians are too often run ragged by people who should worry less about their own health and should be more concerned about what to do with the relatively good health they already possess.

II. *Diversify your diet.* The advice to avoid worry does not preclude the use of intelligent care. Diversification of diet means, of course, substantial diversification; selection should be made from different *types* of food. Some diversification is involved if one includes in one's diet corn, beans, rice, and buckwheat cakes. But such diversification is inadequate because all these are seed products and thus belong in the same general category. A much wider diversification is possible when one considers the following types of foodstuffs: (1) milk and dairy products; (2) seed (including nut) products; (3) meats (not exclusively muscle) from mammals and fowls; (4) fish and marine products; (5) leafy (green) vegetables; (6) root and tuber vegetables, including carrots and potatoes (yellowness is associated with a source of vitamin A); (7) fruits of all kinds, including melons and tomatoes; (8) fungi—yeast, mushrooms, truffles; (9) eggs.

No one should feel under obligation to sample all these foods every day or every month; they are listed merely to indicate that a wide range exists from which to choose. Some people's idea of an excellent meal (to be repeated as often as feasible) is a selection of steak or prime rib roast, baked or French fried potatoes, a dab of salad (mostly for looks), and topped with coffee and, to avoid extra calories, perhaps a little sherbet rather than a heavier dessert like ice cream. Such people need to have their eyes opened to the facts of diversity and to the listing given above. If one selects widely from the types of food listed above and consumes substantial proportions of many of these, the chances of getting a well-balanced diet is vastly greater than if one merely repeats meals like the one described above.

Several of the foods included in the types listed above are by nature relatively well rounded; milk is what nature has provided as a complete food for young; oysters and clams are substantially whole organisms, as are also yeast and mushrooms; eggs are in a sense the equivalent of whole organisms. Each of these items carries in itself the equivalent of some substantial diversification.

In spite of the merits of diversification, it is surprising how some individuals can get into a rut in their selection of food and still appear to thrive. Such individuals prove, *if they con-*

tinue to be well, that rules which apply to many, have their exceptions. They also demonstrate the possession of bodily wisdom which tends to supersede all fixed rules.

It is possible that individual adults who appear to eat unwisely (from the standpoint of accepted nutritional standards) and yet live to advanced age in good health, have been unusually well nourished during youth, and that this foundation of good health is sufficiently strong to withstand considerable abuse in later life. Many of our biologically distant relatives, the insects, exhibit this characteristic in their nutritional history; in the larval stage their nutrition may require every mineral, amino acid, and vitamin in the book, but after they become adult, they can live on pure sugar alone! No adult human being (or other mammal) can even approach living on "naked" calories (as can a fly or bee), but some individuals are more able than others to disregard the rules of well-rounded nutrition.

The fact (and it does appear to be one) that some individuals can thrive on relatively monotonous and one-sided diets, tends to make it difficult for the general public to accept at their face value the preachments of nutritionists. The idea that what one individual can do, others should be able to do equally well, is subject to such a multitude of exceptions, however, that we should not be surprised by one more. Unless my reader is a superman or superwoman and has already demonstrated that he or she can live and thrive on a one-sided diet, the advice to diversify is, I feel sure, good and wholesome.

III. *Use and cultivate your body wisdom.* This advice requires some explanation. We have already mentioned the existence of appetite-regulating mechanisms that help us decide how much to eat, how much water to drink, how much sugar and how much fat to eat, how much salt to use. Mechanisms also govern our appetite for lime (calcium), phosphate, and probably a considerable number of other essential nutrients. These appetite mechanisms have not been studied extensively (or intensively) partly because they are so un-uniform from individual to individual, that general conclusions are difficult.

It is probable that these appetite-controlling mechanisms are *exceedingly important* in helping us get what we individually need in our food. If they were all abolished, our lives would probably soon be snuffed out one way or another. In the case of individuals who have lived to advanced age without ever having given nutrition any study or followed any rules of good nutrition, their superior body wisdoms have probably turned the trick. That people do differ in their body wisdoms is apparent from the fact that some people tend to eat and drink unwisely to their own ruination while others have no difficulty whatever avoiding these excesses.

As we have already suggested, superior body wisdom as possessed by an adult, probably has as a foundation excellent nutrition during the period of youth. It is also interesting that many of the men and women who have lived to an advanced age, tend to be somewhat eccentric; they are the kind of people who eat what they want to eat, and are not easily forced by social pressures to follow the questionable customs of others.

There is evidence to indicate that our human bodies adapt to some degree to the nutritional situations with which they are confronted. How great this adaptation is, is not known and it seems unsafe to depend on this means of survival especially when we can choose the other alternative—excellent nutrition.

Part of what is suggested by the phrase "use your body wisdom" involves showing a certain amount of independence and choice in the selection of food. When one, for politeness or for other reasons, always eats whatever is set before him, regardless and without discrimination, he is not using his body wisdom. When one knows and feels that one has had enough, and yet continues to eat just to be sociable or to please the hostess, one is not using his body wisdom. When one eats so much as to give one distress at night, and does not pay attention to the warning and repeats the performance the next time one has a chance, one is not using his body wisdom. If some individuals persist in eating foods and consuming drinks that produce headaches, sleeplessness, or cause other discomfort, they are not using their respective body wisdoms.

If the general public (including hostesses) were educated to the point that everyone could eat, without embarrassment or social pressure, exactly what their body wisdom told them to eat, everyone's nutrition would probably be substantially improved. This would not work for those whose appetite mechanisms are already seriously deranged, nor would I imply that body wisdom should be expected to supersede common sense.

The question: how to *cultivate* one's body wisdom (particularly with respect to eating), is one about which we have relatively little direct knowledge. We do know, however, that *good nutrition builds body wisdom,* so one way to cultivate better body wisdom is to follow more closely the accepted rules of good nutrition. Anything that promotes good health, such as plenty of sleep, and a wholesome attitude toward life (good mental hygiene), probably also helps our appetite mechanisms to work better and improves our chances of getting exactly the kinds of food we need.

There is much suggestive evidence, which is accumulating as the years go by, to indicate that consistent moderate exercise, especially of a recreational nature, is an *important way* of improving one's body wisdom. The rationale behind this idea involves the fact that exercise stimulates the circulation of the blood, and thus causes the blood to bring better nourishment (and oxygen supply) to all the tissues, including those that are concerned in regulating appetite. Mental relaxation does things to us chemically, and improves our bodily functioning. It is a fact that people who exercise freely, consistently, and enjoyably, day after day, month after month, and decade after decade, are not troubled with obesity; their appestats which govern how much they eat, do not tend to become deranged.

Dean Roscoe Pound, Harvard nonagenarian, who wrote a five-volume work on American jurisprudence between the ages of 86 and 89, is said to have walked thousands of miles all over Scotland, Ireland, and France. In his earlier years he participated in many extensive bicycle trips.

Alonzo Stagg, at 98, still mowed his own lawn and did not indulge himself even to the extent of using a power mower. Thomas Jefferson, who lived to be 83, was a strong advocate of walking and decried the use of horses for transportation. He would certainly be shocked if he were alive today, at the lack of sidewalks in so many localities and the inordinate use of automobiles even for journeys into the next block. Some old-fashioned people today, decry the use of golf carts in a game that is played at least partly for the exercise of walking. Personally, I think that this means of locomotion for the aged and for those whose heart or other condition might be damaged by too much exercise, is justified and wholesome, but when healthy young men and women use this means to avoid exercise, it is not a wholesome sign. Avoidance of moderate exercise is not the way to build up one's body wisdom. In fact, in some quarters there is advocacy of vigorous exercise (properly controlled) as a treatment for heart disease.

Paul Dudley White, the famous heart specialist, is a strong advocate of exercise and he, himself, in a day when in America this means of locomotion is somewhat outmoded, often rides a bicycle, somewhat to the consternation of his more modern contemporaries. Bertrand Russell, the famous philosopher, at age 88, said that our happiness depends on our physiology more than we wish to admit and that unhappy businessmen would benefit more from walking six miles a day than by any change in philosophy.

It is possible that our vexing parking problems and the

consequent increased use of bicycles by college students, for example, are in reality not a curse but a blessing.

Thomas Parr in England, one of the longest-lived men in recorded medical history (1483–1635), was accustomed to thresh grain at the age of 130 and continued to be active until his death at 152. He lived under nine British kings and a monument to his memory is in Westminster Abbey. In view of the known relationships between exercise, obesity, and longevity, the fact seems to be inescapable that sedentarianism is crippling many lives today. It may be very humorous when Robert Hutchins says that he overcomes the urge to exercise by taking a nap, but it is not funny when millions of Americans follow his example, and thereby lose their health, vigor, and part of their body wisdom.

One unfortunate aspect of this situation is that some individuals seem to *hate* to exert themselves physically. They are liable to take the attitude "I may not live as long, but I'm going to be comfortable as long as I do live." Whether there is any cure, nutritional or otherwise, for this situation I do not know. This is indeed a free country. I cannot help feeling that the person who *likes* to be active is a most fortunate one.

It seems probable that one of the reasons why women live longer than men is because they tend to exercise more consistently. "Woman's work is never done"; they probably tend to be on their feet more than men, and do not so often try to make up for days of relative inactivity by periodically indulging in violent exercise.

IV. *Avoid too much refined food.* By refined food is meant refined sugar, alcohol, highly milled rice, and to a lesser degree, products made from white flour, even though it is "enriched." Enrichment of white flour and bread which was initiated about twenty years ago, was an important practical step to bring better nutrition to the public by returning to the flour some of the vitamins and minerals lost in milling.

This was only a partial expedient, as every advocate of enrichment realized, and the procedure should be subject to periodic review and improvement. It has not been kept up to date.

Parenthetically, some readers may need to be reminded that in the highly organized society we live in there are terrific problems of food transportation and storage to be considered as well as potent and compelling human tastes and customs to be dealt with. It is all very well to say to Oriental people "Do not polish your rice," but it is virtually impossible to store any other kind of rice in the tropics, and even the lowliest Oriental laborer prefers clean white rice to brown rice infested with weevils and vermin. When and if ways are found to store and ship whole-wheat flour economically and make products from it that will be generally acceptable, the use of enriched white flour can be terminated. However, the visionaries who imagine that white flour is merely a silly invention of the devil have much to learn about the problems of food production, storage and marketing in a complex society.

In view of the advice "avoid too much refined food," the question arises: "How much is too much?" Students of nutrition would not all agree on the same answer though they would agree that for children the restrictions on refined foods should be relatively severe. When a child (or even an adult) substitutes a soft drink (which is mostly sugar-water) for milk as a mealtime beverage, this is a serious breach of good nutritional sense.

The basic reason why we should avoid excessive refined foods may be explained by an analogy to an outboard motor which is designed so that the fuel and the lubricant (oil) are put together in the same tank. The fuel makes the engine go; the lubricant keeps it in condition. The fuel which we human beings consume is carbohydrate, protein, and fat; while the minerals, vitamins, and essential amino acids may be likened to lubricants. The enzymes into which they enter are, in a fundamental sense, lubricants as we have indicated; they lubricate chemical reactions and allow them to take place rapidly at moderate temperatures.

The common recommendation for an outboard motor is one quart of oil to five gallons of gasoline. One who has an outboard motor could experiment, if he wished, with skimping on the lubricant. Instead of one quart to five gallons, he could try three fourths of a quart or even a pint. While the engine is new it will doubtless run, even if one pint of oil is used. What would be saved on oil would, however, be lost a hundred times over in the deterioration of the motor.

When we consume essentially refined fuel—sugar, alcohol, refined foods—we crowd out of our diets the vital lubricants: amino acids, vitamins, and minerals. With established exercise habits, we consume a specific number of calories per day or per week, and when we consume one half of our calories in the form of lubricant-free food, we are in effect substituting one pint of oil for the recommended quart. If one fourth of our food is lubricant-free and the rest excellent, we are substituting a pint and a half for a quart.

There is one kind of "counting calories" that I would recommend: namely, counting the lubricant-free, or naked, calories from the refined foods you eat. If the total amounts to as much as 600 calories per day, this suggests you are skimping on your lubricants to the extent of about one fourth, even though all the rest of your food is of the highest quality and perfectly chosen. It is estimated that in the U.S.A. and Canada, about one quarter pound of sugar per day per person is consumed on the average. This in itself accounts for about 500 calories. Everyone, of course, is entitled to skimp on lubricants as much as he pleases or as much as he thinks safe. My advice is: *watch it*. Below is given a table designed to help you count your naked, or lubricant-free, calories.

Foods Which Yield Calories Almost Exclusively

Sugar, 1 oz. (2 tablespoons)	100 Cal.
(This is often hidden in foods prepared for the table, especially in desserts.)	
Hard candy, one small piece	10 Cal.
Fudge 2″ × 2″ × ⅝″	185 Cal.
Syrup—1 tablespoon	50 Cal.
Honey—1 tablespoon	85 Cal.
(This is good food for bees (p. 95) but is almost exclusively sugars.)	
Soft drink, 6 oz.	85–150 Cal.
Soft drink, 12 oz.	170–300 Cal.
Soft drink, 12 oz. (sugarless)	6 Cal.
Whiskey, 1½ oz. jigger	120 Cal.
Soft drink, 6 oz., plus 1½ oz. whiskey	205–270 Cal.
Beer, 12 oz.	145 Cal.
(This is not quite free from lubricants but is far from balanced.)	

Foods (for comparison) Which Yield Calories plus Lubricants

Egg, one	75 Cal.
Butter or margarine 1″ × 1″ × ½″	80 Cal.
(Fats yield abundance of calories but these contain highly unsaturated fat acids and vitamin A also.)	
Milk, half pint	170 Cal.
Skim milk, half pint	90 Cal.
Ice Cream, ¼ pint	190 Cal.

For adults, the importance of avoiding refined foods varies from individual to individual. If an adult is hale and hearty in every way and has been using refined foods for decades, I would have no basis for suggesting a change except possibly because of approaching ills associated with aging. On the other hand, if one has health problems particularly related to the material discussed in Chapter V of this book, then I think the admonition to avoid excessive refined foods is important. In another book I have advised alcoholics, who have a severe nutritional problem, to avoid refined foods as completely as possible.

Individuals who are highly active physically can probably tolerate more refined food than others. Because of their activity they use up more calories, this means they eat more food, and have a better chance of getting enough of the lubricants they need. In an earlier society, made up largely of active farmers, good nutrition was easier to maintain partly for this reason.

The use of large amounts of processed foods is not recommended for those who have reason to be seriously concerned about their nutrition. Prepared foods are often toasted which tends to destroy at least one of the potentially important vitamins (p. 118). Processed foods are often claimed to have various specified percentages of those nutrients which the Food and Drug Administration has recognized as established needs, but no attention is paid to other nutrients which informed experts know are also necessary. If we could gather our oranges, apples, carrots, wheat, lettuce, oysters, eggs, fish, pork, and beef, etc., in our own backyards, process them ourselves when necessary and eat them in the fresh state, this might be ideal. Not everything we like grows in the same locality in the same season, however, but fortunately the use of frozen foods and modern transportation makes it possible for us to get great variety.

Canning is also an invaluable expedient, and modern canning preserves a large part of the food value of everything that is canned. Vitamin C, for example, is destroyed by a combination of heat and air (oxygen). In modern canning, the air is excluded and the vitamin C is preserved. There is, however, some sense to the maxim "Eat some raw food every day," because there may be "unknowns" that are altered or destroyed by cooking. Cooking with plenty of water and then discarding the water is a bad practice since substantial amounts of minerals and vitamins are lost.

V. *Use nutritional supplements when, on the basis of informed opinion, it seems desirable.* There are two reasons for using nutritional supplements: first, to combat ailments of the various kinds discussed in Chapter V, including illnesses associated with aging. Parts of our working machinery tend to wear unequally as we age, and the use of supplements may cancel or diminish the difficulties which result. The treatment of disease or illness should be in the hands of a physician.

The second reason for using nutritional supplements involves *insurance* against all ills which may have a nutritional basis. While one may be well and give promise of remaining so, a prudent person provides for the "ifs" of life. No one can be sure, especially if refined foods are used, that he will never be affected adversely by deficient nutrition.

It is for this reason that many reasonably healthy people use nutritional supplements regularly. There is room here for individual preference and judgment. Whether we like it or not, trivial matters such as aversion or liking for "pills," enter into people's decisions. Their financial circumstances and their thrift with respect to such expenditures also play a part. People are notoriously inconsistent in their expenditures. Some would not hesitate a moment to spend several dollars for a good steak or a bottle of liquor, but would shrink from the expenditure of a similar amount for several months' supply of a nutritional supplement—even though it might constitute cheap health insurance.

There are two groups of people who have acute difficulties clearly associated with nutrition and who may be given special advice. These include those with an overweight problem and those who suffer from food allergies.

Overweight is a serious health problem and unfortunately no one knows how to handle it effectively. Good advice is: Try any and every nutritional measure consistent with common sense. Some of the measures may help in your individual case. The use of chemical agents of Type I (p. 86) should be avoided. Physicians are not likely to prescribe them, and certainly they should not be taken otherwise.

The crux of the problem (if you have one) involves getting your appetite-regulating machinery in working order so that you eat just as much as you should and no more. But, how to do it! The idea that people should count their calories and stop when they have had enough sounds fine, but it is an idea that usually doesn't work, except perhaps in mild cases. Usually laymen count their calories incorrectly, for one thing, but more important than this, the fundamental difficulty is not one of *ignorance* about exactly when to stop eating. People who have a weight problem, like everyone else, do not *want* to stop eating while they are still hungry. If they could do this consistently they would avoid obesity. While people who tend to be overweight sometimes follow such a program for a time, sooner or later they revert.

Instead of trying to keep rigid books on how many calories one eats, a person with a weight problem should watch his weight day by day—this will tell the story. Of course there is no merit in being ignorant about calories. Some foods—fresh vegetables, for example—contain a high percentage of water. These contain relatively very few calories per ounce or pound compared with the solid, relatively dry, foods. Fatty foods, on a water-free basis, contain about twice as many calories per pound as do foods which are predominantly protein and carbohydrate calculated in the same manner. If these facts are remembered and acted upon and one's weight is watched carefully, greater benefits will accrue than if one tries to figure out exactly how many calories he consumes each day. Even small differences (p. 51) in the tendency to assimilate foods, could make one individual obese and the other lean, even though they consumed exactly the same number of calories and exercised the same amount. The balance between the assimilated food and the burning-up process in the body is the crux of the problem.

Whenever I think of reducing diets it brings back the memory of a former colleague, long since deceased, who weighed about 300 pounds. He was on a "900-calorie diet" because of his obesity. I saw him go into a drugstore in midmorning, take three cups of coffee with plenty of cream in each, and come out munching from a large bag of shelled peanuts which he carried as a reserve. I think he knew he wasn't playing the game fair. Anyway he had a sense of humor. As he walked out of the drugstore he encountered a corpulent, lazy dog lying on the doorstep. As he pushed him aside he said with conviction, "Pooch, you are too fat."

Much that has been said about cultivating body wisdom applies to the weight problem, and every expedient suggested in that connection deserves serious trial: (1) following the rules which will yield extra good nutrition; (2) exercising regularly and moderately; (3) getting enough sleep and observing good mental hygiene. Included in the rules of good nutrition are the diversification of one's diet, the avoidance of too much refined food, and the possible use of nutritional supplements. The problem of treating obesity involves so many human variables that no one has demonstrated that these expedients will substantially help obese individuals, but there is every reason to think that they will, if applied persistently and intelligently.

I cannot become wildly enthusiastic about the efficacy of Metrecal and similar products as a solution to the weight problem. If they continue to help obese individuals without introducing new troubles, well and good. Nothing succeeds like success.

The use of Metrecal or any similar preparation as a sole article of diet over a long period of time is not recommended; first, because it does not have the advantage of a highly diversified diet. While such preparations may have in them everything that the Food and Drug Administration recognizes as essential, they may lack sufficient amounts of other items that expert biochemists know are also needed. Second, experience and an insight into how nutrition works both indicate that *no single mixture* is likely to be continuously an acceptable food for all members of the human population. If any of my readers have found benefit in Metrecal or similar products, I would not suggest leaving it alone. I would suggest (but I doubt if the suggestion is really necessary) that it not be your sole article of diet, week after week and month after month.

Recently a modified cellulose preparation (Amvicel) has been developed that can be incorporated into salad dressings, desserts, etc., which, it is claimed, has the effect of satisfying hunger without furnishing calories. If this material works out, if it succeeds in fooling the appetite mechanism of the body sufficiently to help people, then I am for it. I am suspicious, however, that there will ever be a real solution to the overweight problem until we can bring back health to appetite-regulatory mechanisms which are often very little out of adjustment (p. 51).

The use of saccharin and similar artificial sweeteners has the advantage that they tend to satisfy one's sweet tooth without contributing naked calories. These substances are foreign to the body and for this reason their use is not ideal; they are used in such tiny amounts, however, that any risk involved is small. They may help an individual who has a weight problem to get a more adequate diet—this is important in promoting healthy appetite mechanisms—but they do not satisfy hunger or act as a substitute for calories.

One of the factors that affects one's appetite is smoking. Many times a person may gain weight when he or she stops smoking, and lose it again when smoking is resumed. Presumably nicotine poisons the appetite mechanism in such a way as to decrease the desire for food. If one chooses to hold one's weight down by smoking, there is no law that prevents one from exercising this choice. It is possible that drugs (remedial chemicals of Type I) will be found that will decrease appetite as the use of tobacco apparently does. I do not have great faith, however, in such expedients. It seems better to strive toward means of making appetite-regulating mechanisms healthy so they will not need to be clubbed into submission.

There may be among my readers those who are suffering from food allergies; in some cases they may not be aware of it. It is an accepted fact that some people become allergic to milk proteins or wheat proteins or egg proteins, etc.—as a result they suffer from many types of difficulties unless they scrupulously avoid the offending foods.

One physician, the late Dr. Arthur F. Coca, was convinced that food allergies are very commonplace and are the hidden cause of many diseased conditions not usually associated with allergies. He also claimed that foods one was allergic to could be spotted by carefully watching one's pulse and by noting which foods caused an increase in pulse rate. His enthusiasm bordered on the extreme, however, and very few physicians take his ideas seriously. When and if "pulse meters" become available so that keeping a record of one's pulse will not be so bothersome, it may be possible that this may be a means of avoiding those food allergies which are at present obscure.

Those who are subject to food allergies are advised to find out with the help of a physician what foods to avoid, and then plan food consumption so that, in spite of the certain lacks, the diet is still well diversified. Since allergies cause stress within one's body, a good supply of the dietary essentials is desirable to take care of the increased needs. All of the nutritional expedients suggested, including the possible use of dietary supplements, should be considered in dealing with allergic conditions.

IX

Nutritional Supplements

The fundamental basis for using nutritional supplements is first, to *treat* the numerous diseases which may have a nutritional basis, including those involved in aging; and second, to *prevent* or to serve as *insurance* against these same diseases.

The treatment of disease should be in the hands of experts —the physicians who are trained in reputable medical schools and know thousands of things about the treatment of disease that lay patients cannot know. Anyone who fails to get medical help when illness overtakes him is foolish and is performing a disservice to his country.

The prevention of disease is, however, on a somewhat different basis. It is the duty of every citizen to be informed about health measures, to observe rules of sanitation, to eat wisely, and to prevent disease whenever he can. If, on the basis of the best expert opinion he can get (not, advisedly, from a salesman), a citizen buys insurance for himself or family against various ills in the form of nutritional supplements, he is carrying out a normal activity.

Nutritional chemicals (belonging in Type II, p. 86) have always been available to the public without prescription. If anyone has reasons for believing that he would be benefited by the use of these agents, he is at liberty to make a trial. He may even draw a false conclusion from his trial: he may decide that he has been benefited by their consumption when actually the benefit has resulted from wishful thinking or self-suggestion. It is a recognizable and undeniable fact that some individuals are highly suggestible—the same ones are also relatively easy to hypnotize—with the result that if a convincing, persuasive individual gives them a sugar pill with the proper incantations, it is likely to bring benefit. On the other hand, there are individuals to whom suggestion is relatively ineffective. These are benefited substantially only when the medication has physiological value. It is probable that nutritional quacks—including a very few licensed physicians—make their music pay off largely by reason of those who are easily persuaded.

Inasmuch as I am not a physician and think that the treatment of disease should be in the hands of experts—the physicians—I will not presume to formulate or discuss any nutritional supplement which has for its purpose the treatment of any disease. Rather I will deal with supplements designed to prevent, or to serve as insurance against all those diseases that may have a nutritional origin.

When one buys insurance, it should be *good* insurance if this can be obtained. Millions of people are at the present time spending a few hundred million dollars annually for nutritional insurance—most often of poor quality and often unduly high priced. The quality of the nutrients used is in general satisfactory but the compounding is very frequently at fault. One of the important purposes of this little book is to point out how the quality of this nutritional insurance can be greatly improved.

On purely logical grounds, a supplement designed as nutritional insurance might contain a balanced assortment of every essential nutrient that humans need. This is entirely impractical, however, because the amino acids, for example, are needed in gram quantities, and to supply a single day's ration of each would cost many dollars and the bulk would be large and the mixture unappetizing. Some of the minerals—

calcium and phosphate are examples—are also needed in approximately gram quantities and any significant supplement is certain to be bulky. Such nutrients as the amino acids, unsaturated fat acids, and the major minerals must ordinarily be obtained from the food we eat. The use of nutritional supplements is not a substitute for sensible eating.

The ingredients of a useful general supplement must, on a practical basis, be largely those nutrients that are needed in small amounts and can be combined in capsules or tablets that can be sold reasonably and administered readily. This limits the included nutrients mostly to vitamins (and related compounds) and to trace minerals. This limitation is not too severe in that there are over 20 essential nutrients that can, without too much difficulty and without inordinate expense, be introduced into supplements.

Formulated below is a nutritional supplement which constitutes, for the general public, a far better package of insurance than any commonly used formulation. For practical reasons the items are placed in two groups, the vitamins and the minerals.

Other chemical items that deserve some consideration as nutritional supplements (at least in special cases) include: (1) folic acid (see p. 119), (2) rutin and related glucosides which have been recommended (on the basis of *un*satisfactory evidence) for capillary weakness and prevention of hemorrhage; (3) glutamine (in *gram* quantities) for help in the prevention of stomach ulcers, alcoholism, and epileptic seizures; (4) asparagin and/or salts of aspartic acid (in gram quantities) for possible benefit in increasing stamina, etc.; (5) lysine (in gram quantities) which markedly supplements the value of many vegetable proteins; (6) lipoic acid, one of the newer vitaminlike substances to be discovered; (7) lecithin which furnishes phosphate and choline and may have other advantages; (8) the "intrinsic factor" which with B_{12} protects against pernicious anemia. This is not an exhaustive list, since additional amino acids and other physiologically important substances may have some value in particular instances. The use of unfamiliar supplements—those which are not now used —may be around the corner.

VITAMINS			MINERALS‡		
Vitamin A	10,000	units	Calcium	300	mg.
Vitamin D	500	units	Phosphate	250	mg.
Ascorbic acid	100	mg.*	Magnesium	100	mg.
Thiamin	2	mg.	Cobalt	0.1	mg.
Riboflavin	2	mg.	Copper	1.0	mg.
Pyridoxin	3	mg.	Iodine	0.1	mg.
Niacinamide	20	mg.	Iron	10.	mg.
Pantothenate	20	mg.	Manganese	1.0	mg.
Vitamin B_{12}	5	mcg.*	Molybdenum	.2	mg.
Tocopherols			Zinc	5.	mg.
(Vit. E.)	5	mg.			
Inositol†	100	mg.			
Choline	100	mg.			

* 1 gram = $\frac{1}{28}$ oz.
  1 milligram (mg.) is $\frac{1}{1000}$ of a gram
  1 microgram (mcg.) $\frac{1}{1,000,000}$ of a gram
† Many nutritionists will assert justifiably that this item has not been proven to be a nutritional essential. It is included, however, on a somewhat different basis (See below).
‡ Some of the items and the proportions indicated may require adjustment due in part to possible restrictions which are under consideration by the Food and Drug Administration.

The rationale behind nutritional insurance is to supply not only the items which are most likely to be helpful but also items that are only possibilities, provided they are not too expensive and are known to be harmless. In buying fire insurance one wants general coverage, not coverage only for those fires arising from causes which the experts regard as important. There is accordingly included in the supplement as formulated, one item (inositol) which is not known to be essential in human diets; in the writer's judgment, partly on the basis of unpublished findings with which he is acquainted, its inclusion is wise even though it may be argued that the chance of its being helpful is relatively low. Vitamin A is at levels higher than is often recommended. This has a reason behind it, because in the author's judgment there are people (perhaps 10 per cent or less) who have requirements much higher than those of the general population. This insurance is for them, too.

Like fire insurance which we buy hoping never to need, nutritional insurance for many individuals who eat wisely may be entirely unnecessary. Nevertheless the opportunities to buy good rather than inferior nutritional insurance should be available.

The most important considerations of all in connection with formulating such a supplement are *quantitative* ones; the amounts indicated are those suggested for daily use. If these amounts are seriously out of balance, as they frequently are in preparations now on the market, they may become worthless in individual cases.

A great deal of care was exercised in deciding upon the amounts to be used. For example, in the case of each item the questions were asked: "How much of it do we need?" "How much of it is in our bodies?" and "Can an extra amount be harmful?" These questions have not been asked in connection with the formulation of many supplements now on the market, including those sold by "old reliable drug houses," and often bearing names that are almost household words.

A group of ten independent druggists was asked individually and anonymously what three vitamin supplements in their judgment were marketed most widely. Their composite ratings were pooled and we shall use Formulation I, Formulation II and Formulation III to designate three of the most widely used brands, containing no minerals. Formulation IV will be used to designate a preparation that contains minerals and which was rated second by two druggists.

Formulation I was rated highest in sales and was lowest

in price. Probably there is a close connection between these two facts. Its value as a nutritional supplement is limited in that it contains no vitamin E, no inositol nor choline, no minerals, and too little vitamin A, vitamin C, pyridoxin, pantothenate, and B_{12} to balance the generous amounts of thiamin and riboflavin that enter into its formulation. People sometimes judge a vitamin mixture by its content of thiamin or B_1 (which is relatively cheap)—a policy which may have been excusable twenty years ago, but not today.

Formulation II is almost twice as expensive as Formulation I, contains about twice as much of some of the vitamins (A, C, D, B_1, B_2 and B_6) but again lacks vitamin E and has a pantothenate level about $\frac{1}{10}$ as high as it should be to balance the levels of B_1 and B_2.

Formulation III is still more expensive; it contains still larger amounts of most of the better known vitamins (including 6 mcg. of vitamin B_{12} as contrasted with 2 mcg. for the others) but it is not conspicuously well balanced and lacks vitamin E, choline, and inositol.

The tendency to apply the principle "if a little is good, more is better" may be observed in connection with these formulations. The more expensive (and hence presumably better) formulations have in general *more of the same*. The formulation I have suggested (p. 112) is not characterized by excessive amounts but by a judicious balance.

Formulation IV containing minerals is about the same price as Formulation III and is similar to it except for the addition of minerals. However, it is much lower in pyridoxin (in proportion to the other ingredients); also, it contains some vitamin E, but not in an amount to balance the relatively high levels of the other vitamins. Inositol and choline are lacking. Six items out of eleven in the mineral supplement are at acceptable levels, three are at relatively low levels, and two, potassium and magnesium, should not have been included and are at ridiculously low levels.

It seems indefensible, as is done in Formulation IV, to supplement a need for magnesium, which is about 250 mg. daily, with a 6 mg. addition. This supplementation could only have propaganda value. Even more ridiculous is the item: 5 mg. of potassium. We ordinarily get in good food something of the order of 2,500 mg. of potassium a day. To supplement this with less potassium than may be derived from a single lima bean is complete nonsense!

All these over-the-counter vitamin preparations have several common defects. Since the public is going to buy them, and the beneficial results to be obtained from their use are individual and hard to evaluate (even though they may in many cases be crucially important), their composition is geared too much to public ignorance and too little to modern scientific knowledge. *Plenty* of certain vitamins (thiamin or vitamin B_1 is an example) are used because they are well known and relatively cheap, and certain other vitamins (such as pyridoxin, or vitamin B_6) are used sparingly because they are not so well known and are much more expensive. I think the reader has adequate basis for realizing that vitamin B_6 is not a *sixth-rate* vitamin simply because it happened to get the number "6" attached to its name! For individual cases it may be the most important vitamin supplement in the lot.

The insignificant supplementation of magnesium and potassium referred to in connection with the discussion of Formulation IV is an example of catering to public ignorance. To those buyers for whom nutritional items are meaningless names, the larger the number of items, the more impressive is the product. If two preparations are offered for sale—one said to be supplemented in magnesium and potassium, the other not, the buyer is likely to think he is getting more for his money in the former case when actually what he gets is totally insignificant and worthless.

As a result of catering too much to public ignorance, over-the-counter preparations tend to be far out of date. In the sale of television sets, manufacturers are forced to keep up to date because buyers can *see the difference*. In the sale of vitamin supplementation for insurance or promotion of health, the results are far from uniform and are often vitiated by the effects of suggestion; as a result the public can be fooled. If the same mixture is sold for ten or twenty years, during which time phenomenal progress is being made in the field of vitamin biochemistry, the mixture obviously gets out of date. Yet the public will buy for lack of more recent information.

Physicians often advise convalescent or other patients to take "a multivitamin preparation" daily without specifying any particular brand. Even the more widely used brands are compounded, as we have seen, without adequate attention to recent advances in nutritional science.

An illustration of this out-of-dateness may be cited from the author's own experience. As the result of the labors of his co-workers and himself for approximately twenty years (about 1920–1940) one of the essential vitamins, pantothenic acid, was discovered and made available to the public. Another twenty years has now passed and very little intelligent use of this vitamin has yet been made in vitamin supplementation for human use. Every biochemist knows that this vitamin is an essential ingredient of coenzyme A, which is an indispensable link in the machinery that lets us get energy from our food; it is necessary for building up of all the essential fatlike components of our bodies as well as many other essential chemicals and for the degradation (tearing down) of all fats.

Recently, however, a supposed expert, writing in a medical journal, has said: "There is little chance of a spontaneous pantothenic acid deficiency in the human diet because of the widespread distribution of this factor in natural foods." This represents a wholly out-of-date point of view, but unfortunately it expresses an idea widely held by those "experts" who are ten to twenty years behind the times.

Twenty or more years ago it may have been presumed that "widespread distribution" was peculiar to pantothenic acid. Now we know that other vitamins for which human deficiencies are well recognized—vitamins B_1, B_2, B_{12} and niacinamide—are widely distributed in the same way that pantothenic acid is.

Whether or not human beings are subject to pantothenic-acid deficiency depends on how their needs compare *quantitatively* with the available supply. Wide distribution, without regard to the quantities, has nothing whatever to do with the question of human deficiencies. The quantitative aspects of nutrition are all important.

In choosing a name for the substance which is now known as pantothenic acid, I took into account one of the striking facts about it—its widespread universal occurrence. The word *pantothenic* is from the Greek, meaning "from everywhere." It was the first vitamin for which such universal occurrence was demonstrated. Since that demonstration, however, it has become clear that the other B vitamins belong in the same boat; they are also universally present.

In one sense the name pantothenic acid is an unfortunate one because it suggests to some that the supply exceeds the demand. Actually this suggestion is unfounded. True, pantothenic acid is universal, but the human need is relatively large, and human deficiency, especially under conditions of stress, is by no means ruled out.

That human needs for pantothenic acid are relatively high is indicated by the following facts: Human milk, food designed by nature for human infants, contains 18 times as much pantothenic acid as thiamin (vitamin B_1). This suggests that infants need about 18 times as much pantothenate as B_1. Human muscle, the most abundant tissue in our bodies, contains 11 times as much pantothenate as vitamin B_1. Human muscle is extraordinary in this regard as will be noted from the following table:

PANTOTHENIC/VITAMIN B₁ RATIOS

Muscle, human	11:1
Muscle, beef	8:1
Muscle, sheep	2:1
Muscle, pork	1:1
Muscle, chicken	7:1
Muscle, salmon	5:1
Muscle, halibut	2:1
Muscle, rat	4:1

Human muscle contains in absolute amount at least twice the amount of pantothenate as the other muscles listed. Pork muscle has about seven times the amount of vitamin B_1, but only half as much pantothenate. All of the pantothenate in our muscles must be supplied by nutrition. Milk and eggs both yield ten times as much pantothenate as vitamin B_1.

This information has been available for twenty years and yet many widely sold supplements contain vitamin B_1 and pantothenate at the same levels! Gross neglect of the quantitative aspects of nutrition is evident. In the supplement we have formulated above for human use, the pantothenate level is ten times that of the thiamin level. This is about as it should be. The possibility of human pantothenate deficiency is increased by the fact that dry heat tends to destroy the vitamin, and toasting of human foods is relatively common.

In the area of animal feeding, which we must touch upon only lightly, we find that nutritional supplementation is more nearly up to date. Here, especially when we are interested in producing meat as cheaply and quickly as possible, the objectives are more definite and the results of nutritional supplementation are more easily measured. It is interesting and very much to the point that about two million dollars' worth of pantothenate is sold each year for vitamin supplementation of animal feed.

If we were to accept the reasoning that wide distribution (regardless of quantities) insures against deficiency we would have to conclude that deficiences cannot exist among animals and that all this money is wasted. Actually those who feed animals know better what they are doing than those who feed humans. It is doubtful whether one could stay in the poultry-raising business today who neglects the use of added pantothenate in feed. It is interesting that in chicken muscle there is a 7:1 ratio (p. 118) of pantothenate to vitamin B_1. The available evidence indicates that human needs for this vitamin may be unusually high compared with those of animals.

Another vitamin that has not been put into currently used supplements at high enough levels is pyridoxin (vitamin B_6). In recent years it has been found, for example, that on the basis of objective tests, certain babies have a need for pyridoxin which is three to four times as great as that of many other infants. In order to take care of those individuals who have relatively high needs, the amount of this vitamin should be *at least* at the same level as vitamin B_1 rather than 1/5 to 1/2 as much, as has been common.

Certain other features of the supplement which we have formulated require special discussion. Folic acid (p. 22) is an essential vitamin, but in recent years it has been found that if it is present in nutritional supplements at a protective level, the individuals taking it may nevertheless develop *pernicious anemia* (due to the lack of utilizable vitamin B_{12}) which goes undetected because the folic acid tends to cover up the existence of this serious disease. To combat pernicious anemia the "intrinsic factor" as well as vitamin B_{12} must be used and the treatment should be in the hands of a physician. In order to obviate this danger and protect the public, the Food and Drug Administration has recently ruled that not more than 0.4 mg. of folic acid should be in a daily dose of a vitamin supplement. Because more than one dose of the supplement we have formulated may be taken daily, we have not included folic acid. This is something that must be obtained in the food. Green leafy vegetables and liver are relatively rich sources.

In the list of twenty-two items included in the supplement formulated on page 112 there are four which are present in amounts that are conspicuously small relative to estimated human needs. These are inositol, choline, calcium, and phosphate. The relatively large bulk (also the cost in some cases) is the important factor that limits these amounts. If a supplement is too bulky and unattractive the end result in individual cases is that it will not be used at all. Striving for a perfect supplement, irrespective of bulk, might of itself defeat the whole purpose of the supplement. Practical considerations such as this cannot be completely neglected.

Every item on the list of nutritional needs (p. 21–23) has been considered in making up this supplement. While there are reasons back of each decision regarding these items, we will not take space to justify all of these decisions. In the case of biotin and vitamin K their exclusion is based upon the fact that they appear to be produced by intestinal bacteria to such an extent that their inclusion would involve a superfluous expense. If antibiotics are being taken, it may not be safe to depend on intestinal bacteria as a source for biotin and vitamin K, because bacterial action is hampered by such medication. The general public is protected from unrestricted use of antibiotics by their unavailability except by prescription—also by their high cost.

One of the notable characteristics of vitamins in general is that no danger is involved if they are used in larger amounts than necessary. Ordinarily they will not be utilized unless they are built into the metabolic machinery, and the metabolic machinery will not absorb a large excess. Of course, if one consistently consumes very large doses of vitamins—a hundred or more times what is needed—there may be some demonstrable bad effects. However, in the case of pantothenate, for example, it has been fed at the rate of 1000 mg. per day to monkeys (this is about 500 times what they need) for six months with no observable effects whatever. Human beings have been given 10 grams per day for a six-week period without bad effects. This is about 1000 times their estimated daily intake (p. 22).

As we have previously noted, some of the minerals that are needed in tiny amounts are highly toxic in much larger amounts. It is partly for this reason that the vitamins are separated from the minerals in the supplement described on page 112. The vitamin dosage may safely be taken by adults twice a day, for example, but the mineral dosage should in safety not be greatly exceeded.

The public needs to be aware in connection with the discussion of vitamins and nutrients generally, of the meaning of the terms *natural, artificial,* and *synthetic.* We have already called attention to the fact that each ingredient of our diet (including water) is a *chemical.* Natural chemicals include all those that enter into the make-up of living animals and plants. Artificial chemicals include those that are foreign to our bodies and to our food. Synthetic chemicals are those produced in the laboratory and may be either natural or artificial.

The production of *natural* pantothenic acid by laboratory means will illustrate the meaning of these terms. First, in our laboratories we found indirect evidence of the existence of the vitamin; second, we separated a small amount of it from large quantities of beef liver; third, we determined its chemical structure and learned how to build it up in the laboratory.

In the second step in this process we produced about 10 milligrams ($\frac{1}{2800}$ oz.) of slightly impure calcium pantothenate from hundreds of pounds of liver at a cost of approximately $20,000. This was the natural vitamin; its complete chemical

structure was determined, including the fact that the molecules were all "right-handed" in their configuration.

It was eventually possible to duplicate these molecules
completely in every respect, so that the laboratory product was
purer. Products which were only slightly different in the arrangement of the atoms were of no use whatever. The "left-
handed" form, for example, is useless.

Pantothenic acid obtained from liver, if pure, contains nothing but molecules built (ultimately by green plants) according to a specified pattern. Pantothenic acid built in the
laboratory contains molecules built on exactly the same pattern. The two products if pure are completely indentical and
cannot be told apart by any means whatever. They can't be
told apart by biochemists (the experts); it should be obvious
that they couldn't be told apart by lawyers, preachers, mer-
chants, plumbers, or anyone else.

The advantage of the laboratory-built (synthetic) product
becomes evident when we compare costs. The wholesale price
of the amount that cost us $20,000 to produce from liver, is
now less than one tenth of one cent! The two products are
exactly the same, except that the cheap product is of superior
purity.

The question may arise whether in the supplement as formulated on page 112 we should not have included an extract
of alfalfa, water cress, yeast, or liver to take care of possible
"unknowns" (yet to be discovered), which such extracts may
contain. A consideration of the all-important quantitative
aspects of nutrition, leads us to the conclusion that such
additions are probably insignificant and worthless.

In the course of my experience with pantothenic acid—
also folic acid which was first concentrated in my laboratory
—and with determining the vitamin contents of a vast array
of plant and animal products, it has become very evident that
vitamins are not to be found in nature in concentrated form.
Many tons of spinach and many hundreds of pounds of liver

were used to get tiny amounts of the vitamins mentioned above. Brewers' yeast is relatively a rich source of thiamin and of pantothenic acid. How much dried brewers' yeast would it take to furnish the amounts of thiamin and pantothenic acid contained in the daily supplement formulated on page 112? About half a pound and one pound respectively! If one is going to consume daily *ounces* of the extract of some relatively rich plant or animal source, he might get enough of some unknown to make a difference. Small amounts such as are commonly used in nutritional supplements are physiologically worthless. The way to get the unknowns into our bodies is to eat good wholesome diversified food. Nutritional supplements should be regarded as *supplements* to help insure good nutrition, not as substitutes for intelligent eating.

Another question often arises. How long must one consume nutritional supplements before benefits may be expected? This question must have an indefinite answer because there are many variables that enter into the problem, including the make-up of the individual involved, and the particular ailments which it is hoped to prevent. In general, "Though the mills of God grind slowly, yet they grind exceeding small." Nutritional effects are often not rapid or dramatic, though in some cases they may be.

If one is buying a nutritional supplement as insurance, then the prudent course is to continue its use indefinitely—as long as the insurance is needed. In investigations with experimental animals, the effects of mild nutritional improvement are not expected to show up within a week or two. Since the time scale for humans is many times longer, no one who takes a nutritional supplement for a period less than several months, should think that he has done anything worthwhile nutritionally. There is a sound basis for thinking that many people appear to get no benefits from nutritional supplements for the simple reason that they *dabble* with them, rather than follow through with a consistent program.

Another question that is often asked, relates to when supplements should be taken in relation to meals. The ideal, which involves the least waste, would be to have them dispersed in the intestinal tract along with the food. How important this time element is in the case of each nutrient, no one knows, but on the basis of our present knowledge, taking supplements at mealtime is recommended, though this is not a crucial point. It is more important that the supplements be actually consumed than that they be taken at any particular time of day.

In conclusion, I would like to stress the fact that I have presented facts and revealed insights that should help every individual who is interested in nourishing his or her own body more intelligently and effectively. It is my viewpoint that each individual has a substantial responsibility for ordering his own life, including his consumption of food. If each will take advantage of the unity of nature, diversify his food, avoid too much refined food, cultivate body wisdom, and use nutritional supplements when informed judgment so dictates, I am sure that better health will be the reward.

X

Personal Postscript

If I had written this book about ten years earlier—containing as it does many allusions to the use of pantothenic acid, and an advocacy of its use in nutritional supplements in much larger amounts—my motives might have been suspect.

The discovery of the existence of pantothenic acid was the result of years of work supported mainly by the universities with which I was associated. The initial production of about 10 mg. of calcium pantothenate was supported largely by the Rockefeller Foundation, so that it was never regarded as a purely private venture.

When patents were applied for in connection with the synthesis of the vitamin, no one knew whether, or to what degree, the substance would be useful. These patents were assigned to Research Corporation, a nonprofit organization which supports research. Three fourths of the royalties over which I might have had some control were plowed back into scientific research. The other fourth was divided about equally between my associates and myself.

The reason I can now write freely about pantothenic acid and the advantages of including relatively large amounts of it in nutritional supplements, is that the patents have about run out, and nothing that I can write at this date will make any substantial difference in the royalties I may receive from that source. Scientists must avoid even the appearance of being biased financially, if their opinions are to carry much weight. So I repeat what I said in the preface with added meaning, "The time has come . . . to tell the story of nutrition." I could not have told the story earlier with effectiveness because it could have been said that I was "promoting" pantothenic acid for personal gain.

Of course the material in this book dealing with pantothenic acid is a minor part as I think every reader will recognize. However, the pantothenic-acid material is there and critics would surely have magnified its significance if the book had been written earlier.

Now, however, the full story insofar as pantothenic acid is concerned can be told without fear of this criticism; the public is entitled to know.

1

How to Keep Up to Date
on Nutrition

We have pictured nutrition as a rapidly developing science and have indicated that new information and insights can be expected in the years ahead. How can one keep up with what is being learned?

People who are not in scientific work have little realization of how much is going on day by day and year by year in the world of science. One of the best indications is the scope of one of the largest abstract journals in the world, *Chemical Abstracts*. The many contributors to this journal read articles describing original investigations (as reported in all languages) and prepare a short summary of the contents of each for publication in *Chemical Abstracts*. The total number of magazines (weeklies, monthlies, quarterlies) abstracted is about 8,000; the total number of issues examined per year must be about 80,000 and the abstracts (usually short), in 1960, occupied over 13,000 large double-column fine-print pages.

These abstracts cover the entire field of chemistry and only a fraction of these articles have anything to do with nutrition. This gives a hint, however, as to how extensive the literature of chemistry is. It is a hopeless task, of course, for one to read about all the original work that is done. Even to read the abstracts in a particular field is a big undertaking. Fortunately

Chemical Abstracts, which can be consulted in any larger library, is well indexed each year and each decade.

For most readers, consultation of the abstracts of detailed articles would be too exacting. Fortunately there are other journals, of which *Nutrition Reviews* (The Nutrition Foundation, Inc., 99 Park Avenue, New York 16, New York, $4.00 per year) is outstanding, that seek to "skim the cream" from recent nutritional investigations and present discussions regarding it. Another less-pretentious magazine is a bimonthly, *Borden's Review of Nutrition Research*, available from The Borden Company, 350 Madison Avenue, New York 17, N.Y. Contrary to what might be supposed by laymen, this journal is quite uncontaminated by any propaganda about dairy products. If this were not so, reputable scientists would not write for the journal year after year.

If one is seriously interested in a study of nutrition, he may find references (in *Chemical Abstracts*, for example) to numerous other sources where digests of recent work are presented. One of these is the *Annual Reviews of Biochemistry* (Annual Reviews, Inc., Palo Alto, California, price, $7.00) which presents discussions of various topics and cites references to perhaps 4,000–5,000 new, separate articles each year. A substantial proportion of these have some connection direct or remote to nutrition.

The close connections between biochemistry and nutrition can hardly be exaggerated. No one can be an expert in nutrition without having basic training and insight in chemistry and biochemistry. If any young student aspires to be competent in the field of nutrition, chemical and biochemical study is a *must*.

Of course there are also books on nutrition. One of the best older books for semipopular reading is that of H. C. Sherman, *The Nutritional Improvement of Life*, (Columbia University Press, 1950). Perhaps it seems strange to refer to this as an older book since it is only a little over 10 years old.

Nutrition is indeed a rapidly advancing science and in addition this work was written by Dr. Sherman after he had retired from active work, and presents a somewhat older viewpoint than the date indicates. In its essentials, however, it is eminently sound.

Another book of about the same vintage as Sherman's, *Nutrition in Relation to Health and Disease* (Milbank Memorial Fund, 1950), gives reports and discussions of a number of nutritional experiments mostly involving human beings, and presents some striking evidence as to the importance of adequate nutrition in preventing disease.

One recent book that may be noted is by Ancel and Margaret Keys entitled, *Eat Well and Stay Well* (Doubleday & Co., Inc., 1959). I am not competent to judge the "cookbook" aspects of this work. Dr. Keys, a competent physiologist, is interested primarily in the problems of obesity and heart disease and the book reflects this interest. One would not realize from this book alone that so many other problems of health hinge on good nutrition.

Earlier I have referred to a very recent book (1961) of a more technical nature edited by J. F. Brock, *Recent Advances in Nutrition* (J. & A. Churchill, London). Some of my readers may be sufficiently interested in nutrition to want to peruse this volume. Another valuable book is *The Heinz Handbook of Nutrition* (McGraw-Hill, 1959). This is one of the rare books on nutrition which at least makes a bow (two pages) toward the problem of individuality in nutrition. Norman Desrosier's *Attack on Starvation*, Avi Publishing Company (1961), is another. This devotes a chapter to the subject.

Other authors who have written popularly (or have edited books) on the subject of nutrition in recent years on the basis of professional backgrounds are (alphabetically listed): Ralph W. Gerard now at Michigan; Ruth M. Leverton of the Department of Agriculture, Washington; E. H. McHenry of Toronto; Edmund S. Nasset of Rochester, and Fredrick J.

Stare of Harvard. Books which are solid and dependable are, unfortunately, seldom best sellers.

The author has written two relatively recent books, *Alcoholism: The Nutritional Approach* (University of Texas Press, 1959), and *Biochemical Individuality* (John Wiley & Sons, 1956), both of which deal in part with nutrition. The second book, though technical, has been read with interest by some laymen and has profound implications with respect to individual needs in nutrition.

One of the pitfalls that readers should avoid is the acceptance as truth of opinions on nutrition from those who are primarily *writers* and are only secondhand observers. Even the occasional novelist or movie star who is unenlightened scientifically, sounds off on nutrition and related subjects when he should be listening. Certainly there is an advantage in scrutinizing and *thinking* about what one reads, regardless of who the author may be. Even some formally qualified nutritionists are not sufficiently aware of what has been happening in biochemistry and biochemical genetics in the past ten years to be able to look into the future or even to see the present with a scientific perspective. Biochemistry has advanced tremendously; these advances have *important* implications.

I wish it were possible to give a quick practical answer to the question "What writers on nutrition should we trust most?" Of course there are many competent professional writers who are capable of presenting for public consumption matters of scientific interest. This is all to the good except that some journalistically inclined individuals bring their own inexpert opinions about nutrition into a dominant role. The men or women who are capable of speaking or writing with firsthand intelligence on the subject of nutrition must be trained biochemists and must, in addition, have paid some particular attention to nutrition.

Following is a list of men and women in the U.S.A. who

may be judged competent on the basis of their membership (1960) in *both* the American Institute of Nutrition *and* in the American Society of Biological Chemists. Of course this is not a completely satisfactory list. There are probably some listed who are not particularly competent; others may be omitted who are fully competent but who, for reasons known only to themselves, are not members of both organizations. Membership in the American Society for Clinical Nutrition might also be considered in this connection. Membership or nonmembership in scientific organizations is not an infallible criterion. The list of those who are coincidentally members of *both* organizations—the American Institute of Nutrition *and* the American Society of Biological Chemists —is presented to give the reader concrete evidence that there are hundreds of people more competent professionally to write about nutrition than are those whose writings are followed often with utmost faith. Many of the members of the American Society of Biological Chemists (nearly 1,700 members, carefully screened) have the backgrounds necessary to make valid judgments in the field of nutrition even though their special interests may not be in this area.

MEMBERS (1960)
OF *both* THE AMERICAN INSTITUTE OF NUTRITION *and*
THE AMERICAN SOCIETY OF BIOLOGICAL CHEMISTS

E. H. Ahrens, Jr.
A. A. Albanese
R. B. Alfin-Slater
J. B. Allison
H. J. Almquist
S. R. Ames
W. E. Anderson
C. F. Asenjo
L. Atkin
A. E. Axelrod
C. V. Bailey
R. H. Barnes

C. A. Baumann
E. F. Beach
C. P. Berg
O. A. Bessey
C. H. Best
R. M. Bethke
C. E. Bills
F. G. Bing
F. E. Bischoff
N. R. Blatherwick
R. J. Block
L. E. Booher

A. W. Bosworth
G. M. Briggs
M. Brin
H. P. Broquist
J. B. Brown
H. B. Burch
J. J. Burns
G. O. Burr
W. W. Burr, Jr.
J. S. Butts
F. A. Cajori
M. L. Caldwell
T. M. Carpenter
H. E. Carter
L. R. Cerecedo
J. P. Chandler
V. H. Cheldelin
B. F. Chow
C. L. Comar
J. G. Coniglio
W. E. Comatzer
J. R. Couch
G. R. Cowgill
W. M. Cox, Jr.
F. S. Daft
H. Dam
L. J. Daniel
A. L. Daniels
W. J. Darby
G. K. Davis
H. G. Day
P. L. Day
J. S. Dinning
D. L. Drabkin
R. A. Dutcher
V. du Vigneaud
M. Dye
H. M. Dyer
N. R. Ellis
C. A. Elvehjem
K. Folkers
A. H. Free
T. E. Friedemann
D. V. Frost

C. Funk
M. Goettsch
H. Goss
C. E. Graham
I. Greenwald
W. H. Griffith
C. J. Gubler
N. B. Guerrant
P. György
J. R. Haag
T. S. Hamilton
D. B. Hand
P. Handler
R. G. Hansen
A. E. Harper
P. L. Harris
A. B. Hastings
V. G. Heller
L. M. Henderson
A. G. Hogan
R. T. Holman
J. O. Holmes
L. E. Holt, Jr.
I. M. Hoobler
M. K. Horwitt
E. E. Howe
P. E. Howe
R. B. Hubbell
J. S. Hughes
R. W. Jackson
B. C. Johnson
R. M. Johnson
J. H. Jones
T. H. Jukes
E. O. Keiles
C. Kennedy
J. C. Keresztesy
A. Keys
C. G. King
I. S. Kleiner
W. E. Krauss
W. A. Krehl
H. D. Kruse
A. R. Lamb

A. L. Lehninger
S. Lepkovsky
S. Levey
H. Levine
R. C. Lewis
I. E. Liener
H. E. Longenecker
C. M. Lyman
J. F. Lyman
C. G. Mackenzie
F. L. MacLeod
G. MacLeod
R. MacVicar
F. H. Mattson
L. A. Maynard
W. S. McCann
C. M. McCay
J. F. McClendon
E. V. McCollum
R. H. McCoy
F. G. McDonald
E. W. McHenry
D. Melnick
E. T. Mertz
O. Mickelsen
O. N. Miller
H. H. Mitchell
A. F. Morgan
H. P. Morris
E. H. Mosbach
A. L. Moxon
W. L. Nelson
L. C. Norris
B. L. O'Dell
R. Okey
H. S. Olcott
R. E. Olson
J. M. Orten
H. T. Parsons
P. B. Pearson
J. J. Pfiffner
P. H. Phillips
H. B. Pierce
J. M. Price

F. W. Quackenbush
M. L. Quaife
E. J. Quinn
R. E. Remington
D. A. Richert
T. R. Riggs
D. Rittenberg
J. H. Roe
C. S. Rose
W. C. Rose
F. Rosen
H. R. Rosenberg
S. H. Rubin
W. D. Salmon
L. T. Samuels
I. Sandiford
H. P. Sarett
G. H. Satterfield
H. E. Sauberlich
M. O. Schultze
K. Schwarz
B. S. Schweigert
M. L. Scott
J. V. Scudi
W. H. Sebrell, Jr.
E. L. Severinghaus
R. E. Shank
W. Shive
M. Silverman
S. A. Singal
A. H. Smith
E. E. Snell
H. H. Sobotka
F. J. Stare
G. Stearns
H. Steenbock
J. A. Stekol
E. L. R. Stokstad
L. Swell
M. E. Swendseid
L. J. Teply
H. C. Tidwell
H. W. Titus
W. R. Todd

R. M. Tomarelli   A. White
C. R. Treadwell   J. White
H. C. Trimble   H. H. Williams
B. L. Vallee   J. N. Williams, Jr.
J. van Eys   R. R. Williams
R. Van Reen   E. Woods
H. M. Vars   D. W. Woolley
J. Waddell   L. D. Wright
C. C. Wang

Probably the best basis for judging whether or not to take a person's opinions on nutrition seriously is his or her individual scientific record which can be found in *American Men of Science*, The Jaques Cattell Press, Inc., Tempe, Arizona. As indicated earlier (p. 84) many of the more prolific and supposedly authoritative writers on nutrition have no scientific record and hence cannot rightfully be regarded as authentic spokesmen in this field.

The American Institute of Nutrition consists of individuals who have done research in nutrition and published their findings in reputable scientific journals. It is truly representative of scientific nutrition in this country. There is another organization with an impressive title made up mostly of dentists and doctors who are enthusiastic about nutrition but lack, in my opinion (and that of many others), adequate backgrounds. Their headquarters (and hindquarters too, I think) are on the West Coast. The Nutrition Foundation, Inc. (New York) publishes the valuable *Nutrition Reviews* referred to above and is thoroughly reputable. The National Vitamin Foundation (New York) is a "nonprofit organization for the advancement of knowledge of the nutritional requirements of man and animals in health and disease" and enjoys a sound reputation. There are other so-called "nutrition foundations" and the like, located elsewhere in the country that do not enjoy a reputation for dependability.

An agency which presumes to advise its customers authoritatively on all types of purchases (*Consumer Reports*) indicates in its buying guide issue (December 1961) that only "in very special cases" may supplementary multiple vitamins be useful. The convictions expressed by the writers of this discussion are far too positive and are based, in my opinion, to a considerable degree on inadequate information and a lack of appreciation of many facts which have been set forth earlier in this book.

In advising readers whom they may trust in the field of nutrition, it is not my purpose to be "anti" anyone in particular. I do wish, however, to combat erroneous ideas, regardless of their source.

Some of the wild ideas that are present in the writings of those who lack adequate background go something like this:

Pasteurized milk is no good as a source of calcium because the enzymes that make the calcium available are destroyed. Pasteurized milk is "dead" milk because the enzymes are gone. Milk is homogenized so stale milk can be mixed with fresh.

Such statements and implications as these are based on ignorance. As we have repeatedly pointed out, enzymes as such are not needed in our food. If they are destroyed (denatured) this is a necessary step in getting the amino acids out of them. Milk and dairy products are handled and regulated with great care; homogenization produces a product which I, among millions of Americans, like better. When it is poured from a container it *all* comes out; the cream is not left behind smeared on the bottle or the carton.

Another idea is expressed something like this:

Glucose is an unnatural, cheap, fraudulent, synthetic filler used in foods. It puts an unnatural load on our pancreatic glands and aggravates the diabetic condition.

This thinking is based purely on ignorance. Glucose is the predominant fuel on which our bodies run. We burn up somewhere near a pound of it a day. The amount in our blood at any one time is small (about ⅓ oz. total) but it is replenished continually. It is absolutely essential for the nourishment of our brains and if the level in the blood gets too low we pass into coma. This is identically the same glucose we buy in corn syrup. It happens not to be a synthetic product but it would be just as good if it were. Synthetic glucose would probably cost at least $100.00 per pound. In the case of glucose, the natural product (obtained by digesting starch) is far cheaper.

As is made clear earlier, the nutritional use of glucose or any other sugar without accompanying lubricants tends to promote deficient nutrition. In this respect glucose has the same effect as cane or beat sugar, starch, or honey. Honey has a high percentage of glucose in it, along with fructose (which is no better and no worse physiologically), and practically nothing else. Adult bees can live on it (infant bees cannot) because they can utilize pure fuel (p. 95).

Another idea that prevails among food faddists is to this effect:

Synthetic vitamins are dangerous; we need the natural ones.

This again results from pure ignorance. In some cases, chemists are able to produce in their laboratories the *same* vitamins that are found naturally. In some cases, they find this very difficult or as yet impossible. Chemists know *better than anyone else* when they can do it and when they can't. They have most exacting criteria of identity—criteria that laymen cannot understand, much less criticize.

It is true that chemists do not know yet how to make in the laboratory all of the constituents of natural food. This is one reason why every reputable nutritionist advises people to eat wisely from diversified foods. However, getting the "unknowns," if they still exist, by partaking of a little water cress, alfalfa, or other "herbs" or "royal jelly" is futile because of the *quantitative* aspects of nutrition (pp. 25, 37, 118) which are absolutely crucial and yet so often neglected.

Another idea that is fostered by some cultists whose background knowledge is far too limited may be expressed as follows:

Stay away from all chemical fertilizers.

Unfortunately for the protagonists of this idea there are no other kinds of fertilizers. Spiritual fertilizers, if they exist, will not promote the growth and well-being of plants.

Of course what the advocates of this idea mean is: Use manures, composts, etc., in preference to anything that anyone called a "chemist" has had anything to do with. No one could or should deny the efficacy of manures, etc., as fertilizing agents. On the other hand anyone who damns anything that an expert chemist touches is extremely ignorant. Manures are complex mixtures of chemicals infested with microorganisms that are often beneficial. Soils differ and manures differ, and it does take expertness based on science or empiricism to know how to use them most effectively. Manures can be analyzed, and if they are low in potash or phosphate or nitrogen in relation to the soil on which they are to be used, then the sensible and intelligent thing is to supplement them with the needed element. All of this requires expertness, and simply involves the addition of more chemicals to the ones already present. If manures contained no chemicals, they would be non-existent.

People who would avoid chemicals in fertilizers point to the fact (which is a fact) that chemists do not produce by laboratory means anything that is the exact duplicate of manure. This is due to the fact that manure is an exceedingly complex mixture of chemicals rather than to its possession of any mysterious qualities not possessed by a mixture of chemical substances inoculated with suitable microorganisms. Protagonists of these ideas are also fond of calling attention to the alleged fact that chemists cannot artifically produce sea water in which sea plants and animals can live. It is true that chemists have never duplicated sea water in the laboratory. The fact is that qualified chemists have never tried very hard to do this. They have spent more time, for example, on a project that appeals to them as being more important—making fresh water out of sea water for the benefit of arid regions.

Sea water is an exceedingly complex mixture—the leached-out minerals which have accumulated there for millions of years, represent about every kind of atom known. It is no wonder that it is difficult to duplicate. Incidentally, ocean water the world over does not have the same composition; the "trace elements," for example, are by no means equally distributed in the Atlantic and the Pacific oceans.

The reader who wishes to keep up with advances in nutrition is advised to avoid seeking counsel from poorly prepared individuals who advance such ideas as those illustrated above. It would take too much space to discuss all the wild ideas which "eloquent" people with limited backgrounds entertain. Many of these pertain to the causes of cancer—a favorite subject because even scientists are not yet perfectly clear on this subject. The best advice I can offer is this: If anyone purports to give nutritional advice or announces some nutritional discovery, make him (male or female) show his biochemical credentials.

2

Statement on Addition of
Specific Nutrients to Foods*

Adopted jointly by the Food and Nutrition Board, National Academy of Sciences—National Research Council, and the Council on Foods and Nutrition, American Medical Association, May 1961.

The Recommended Dietary Allowances, first developed by the Food and Nutrition Board of the National Research Council in 1943, specify levels of nutrient intake judged on scientific evidence to be desirable goals for the maintenance of good nutrition of healthy persons in the United States. The recommendations were revised in 1945, 1948, 1953, and 1958, as new data on nutritional needs became available. The nutrients for which allowances are specified and all other essential nutrients for healthful nutrition are expected to be provided by a variety of foods commonly available to the general population. To insure this expectation the judicious addition of specific nutrients to certain processed foods has proved useful. A statement of policy in regard to this practice is desirable for guidance of the public and the food industry.

The Council on Foods and Nutrition of the American Medical Association adopted its policies on proper additions of vitamins and minerals to foods in 1939 and again in 1946.

* While this statement has a conservative leaning (this is to be expected of any statement on which *groups* of experts agree), it nevertheless reflects an attitude of awareness with respect to the dangers of deficient nutrition, and is printed here for this reason.

In 1941 the Food and Nutrition Board likewise adopted a policy on the addition of specific nutrients to foods. These statements of policy were reconsidered jointly by the Food and Nutrition Board and the Council on Foods and Nutrition in 1953, were reaffirmed in principle, and with revision of wording were published jointly as a statement of general policy in regard to the addition of specific nutrients to foods. There is good evidence to indicate that the policies have been beneficial to the public and have encouraged sound nutritional practices during a period of increasing awareness by both producers and consumers of the nutritional and economic problems of supplementation of foods with specific nutrients.

The 1953 statement of general policy has now been reexamined to determine its accuracy, realism, and usefulness in the light of experience and from the viewpoints of existing and probable nutritional needs in the United States, of current and anticipated agricultural production of food in relation to an increasing population, and of prudent application of technological developments in the industrial preparation of nutrients and in the processing of foods. On the basis of these considerations the policies have been revised in part and are embodied in the following statements:

(1) The principle of the addition of specific nutrients to certain foods is endorsed, with defined limitations, for the purpose of maintaining good nutrition in all segments of the population at all economic levels. The requirements which should be met for the addition of a particular nutrient to a given food include (a) acceptable evidence that the supplemented food would be physiologically or economically advantageous for a significant segment of the consumer population; (b) assurance that the food item concerned would be an effective vehicle of distribution for the nutrient to be added; and (c) evidence that such addition would not be prejudicial to the achievement of a diet good in other respects.

(2) The desirability of meeting nutritional needs by the

use of an adequate variety of foods as far as practicable is emphasized strongly. To that end, research and education are encouraged to insure the proper choice and preparation of foods and to improve food production, processing, storage, and distribution so as to retain their essential nutrients.

(3) Foods suitable as vehicles for the distribution of additional nutrients are those which have a diminished nutritive content as a result of loss in refining or other processing or those which are widely and regularly consumed. The nutrients added to such foods should be the kinds and quantities associated with the class of foods involved. The addition of other than normally-occurring levels of nutrients to these foods may be favored when properly qualified judgment indicates that the addition will be advantageous to public health and when other methods for effecting the desired purpose appear to be less feasible.

(4) Scientific evaluation of the desirability of restoring an essential nutrient or nutrients to the diet is necessary whenever technologic or economic changes lead to a nutritionally significant reduction in the intake of a nutrient or nutrients. Such reduction might result either from a marked decrease in the consumption of an important food or from a considerable increase in the consumption of foods of diminished nutritive quality.

Similar evaluation is desirable, with the limitations defined in section (1) above, whenever advances in nutritional science and in food technology make possible the preparation of nutrient-enriched products which are likely to make important contributions to good nutrition.

(5) The endorsement of the following is affirmed: the enrichment of flour, bread, degerminated corn meal, corn grits, whole grain corn meal and white rice; the retention or restoration of thiamin, riboflavin, niacin, and iron in processed food cereals; the addition of vitamin D to milk, fluid skim milk, and nonfat dry milk; the addition of vitamin A to margarine

and to fluid skim milk and nonfat dry milk; and the addition of iodine to table salt. The protective action of fluoride against dental caries is recognized and the standardized addition of fluoride to water is endorsed in areas in which the water supply is low in fluoride.

(6) The above statements of policy and of endorsement apply to conditions existing in the United States. Recommendations for additions of nutrients to foods for export should be based on similar physiological or economic advantages expected to accrue to the respective consumers.

Index

Unity of nature, 33, 37, 38, 79, 88

Universal occurrence, 117

Unsaturated fat acids, 21, 40–41, 46, 49, 58

Unsaturated fats, 49. *See also* Unsaturated fat acids

Uric acid, 50

Vegetarians, 35

Veins, 12

Vigor, 73

Viruslike agents, 64

Visual abilities, 75; pigments, 14–15. *See also* Color blindness

Vitamin supplements. *See also* Nutritional supplements

Vitamin A, 15, 16, 19, 22, 40, 42, 45, 55, 56, 58, 112; deficiency, 10, 41, 55–56

Vitamin B₁ (thiamin), 19, 22, 33, 46, 48, 56, 58, 59, 61, 66, 112, 118; deficiency, 17, 39, 46, 48, 59, 61, 66

Vitamin B₂ (riboflavin), 10, 22, 33, 41, 56, 57, 58, 112; deficiency, 10, 41, 56

Vitamin B₆ (pyridoxin), 22, 33, 46, 47, 57, 58, 62, 115, 119

Vitamin B₁₂ (cobalamin), 22, 33, 41, 46, 57, 59; deficiency, 17, 41, 59

Vitamin C (ascorbic acid), 22, 37, 42, 46, 56, 58, 103, 112; deficiency, 10, 39, 45, 56, 67

Vitamin D, 22, 58

Vitamin E (tocopherols), 15, 16, 22, 40, 45, 58, 112; deficiency, 15, 16, 40

Vitamin K, 22, 46, 120

Vitamins, 22, 26, 27, 33, 34, 38, 53, 83, 100, 101, 112. *See also* Specific vitamins

Water balance, 46

Water cress, extract of, 122

Weight gain, 69

Wernicke's disease, 61

"Wet" beriberi, 46

Whole-wheat flour, 100

Women, longevity of, 99

"Wonderful One Hoss Shay," 55

World population, 80

Worry, 83

Wound healing, 58

Writers on nutrition, 84, 130

Xerophthalmia, 55

Yeast, 94, 122

Zinc, 22, 33, 87; need established, 87

E18